Mental Health Issues and the University Student

Mental Health Issues and the University Student

DORIS IAROVICI, M.D.

Johns Hopkins University Press

BALTIMORE

Note to the Reader. The author has made reasonable efforts to determine that the selection and dosage of drugs and treatments discussed in this text conform to the practices of the general medical community. The medications described do not necessarily have specific approval by the U.S. Food and Drug Administration for use in the diseases and dosages for which they are recommended. In view of ongoing research, changes in governmental regulations, and the constant flow of information relating to drug therapy and drug reactions, the reader is urged to check the package insert of each drug for any change in indications and dosage and for warnings and precautions. This is particularly important when the recommended agent is a new and/or infrequently used drug.

Although the problems and symptoms of students presented in the clinical vignettes in this book are based on frequently encountered symptoms among university students, no vignette describes an actual patient. Names and demographic details are all fictitious; however, they were chosen to reflect patterns encountered in clinical practice.

© 2014 Johns Hopkins University Press
All rights reserved. Published 2014
Printed in the United States of America on acid-free paper
9 8 7 6 5 4 3 2 1

Johns Hopkins University Press
2715 North Charles Street
Baltimore, Maryland 21218-4363
www.press.jhu.edu

Library of Congress Cataloging-in-Publication Data

Iarovici, Doris, author.
  Mental health issues and the university student / Doris Iarovici.
    pages cm
  Includes bibliographical references and index.
  ISBN 978-1-4214-1271-9 (hardcover : alk. paper) — ISBN 1-4214-1271-3 (hardcover : alk. paper) — ISBN 978-1-4214-1238-2 (pbk. : alk. paper) — ISBN 1-4214-1238-1 (pbk. : alk. paper) — ISBN 978-1-4214-1239-9 (electronic) — ISBN 1-4214-1239-x (electronic)
  I. Title.
  [DNLM: 1. Mental Health Services. 2. Universities. 3. Mental Disorders—therapy. 4. Students—psychology. WA 353]
  RC451.4.S7
  616.8900835—dc23   2013021120

A catalog record for this book is available from the British Library.

Special discounts are available for bulk purchases of this book. For more information, please contact Special Sales at 410-516-6936 or specialsales@press.jhu.edu.

Johns Hopkins University Press uses environmentally friendly book materials, including recycled text paper that is composed of at least 30 percent post-consumer waste, whenever possible.

To Ariel and Justin, with love. Wishing you joy and fulfillment in the college years.

Contents

Tables and Figures

PART I / THE STUDENT IN CONTEXT

The Interdependent Campus

CHAPTER 1

Crisis on the College Campus?

College is becoming an aspiration for more and more of America's youth. Nearly half of American 18- to 24-year-olds are enrolled in college at least part-time. With the rise of information technology and an increasingly global economy, higher education is also becoming more of a necessity for success. Although many of us look back fondly on our "bright college years," for growing numbers of students, this is a tumultuous and difficult time. In addition to many normal developmental milestones that can cause emotional challenges, psychiatric disorders often first emerge during these years.

"Record Levels of Stress Found in College Freshmen," trumpeted a headline in the *New York Times* in 2011.[1] Continuing a trend that has been noted since the 1990s, college students were reporting the lowest levels of emotional health in 25 years. This particular finding relied on data from over 200,000 incoming first-year students at four-year colleges across the United States who participated in "The American Freshman: National Norms Fall 2010," the largest and longest-running survey of American college students.[2] The numbers have since remained about the same. In the past decade, many other studies have raised similar concerns about the emotional and mental well-being of students. And it's not just "stress"—depression, anxiety, substance abuse, eating disorders, and other psychiatric issues seem to be on the rise in this population.

Part of the explanation may be that we are getting better at identifying these problems earlier and offering help sooner. More children and adolescents than ever before are receiving effective treatment in high school or earlier for anxiety, depression, and other problems, allowing them to successfully enter college. Some researchers speculate that the trend toward "helicopter parenting," in which parents overmanage every detail of their child's life before college, leads to children whom college deans have called "crispies" or "teacups"—so burned out that they can't engage meaningfully in college life, or so fragile that they break at the first sign of challenge. Admissions officers from selective universities have been speaking out against the craze that pressures families and adolescents to go to extremes in trying to achieve, in order to get into certain colleges. Marilee Jones, a former dean of admissions at the Massachusetts Institute of Technology, teamed up with an adolescent medicine specialist to write the book *Less Stress, More Success*; both authors are concerned that the pressure placed on kids to get into college is actually making them sick.

Regardless of the reasons, those of us who work in college counseling centers can attest to the growing numbers of students we see, as well as to some increase in the complexity and severity of the kinds of problems students bring in. In the most recent National Survey of College Counseling Center Directors, over 90% of directors agreed that the trend toward greater numbers of students with severe psychological problems continues. Increasingly problematic, in the opinion of these directors, are "psychiatric medication issues" and "crisis issues requiring immediate response."[3] And indeed in the last decade, university communities have been buffeted by some emergencies so severe that their effects have reverberated far beyond the campus gates.

Each year of the new millennium seems to bring another high-profile campus tragedy, highlighting unmet mental health needs among college students. There are clusters of suicides, such as the three within a five-week period at New York University in fall 2003, followed by three more that academic year, or the six over a few months in 2009–2010 at Cornell. There have been campus shootings, most notoriously at Virginia Tech in 2007, in which 33 people were massacred, and many others were injured. Sometimes the disasters involve enrolled students; at other times, the perpetrator is a student who was recently dismissed. In retrospect, there were often warning signs of mental distress but a lack of clarity about how best to respond. Jared Loughner, who in January 2011 shot Representative Gabrielle Gifford and 19 others, killing 6, had been suspended from Pima Community College after displaying behavior that was disturbing enough that he was mandated to get a psychological evaluation before he could return to school.[4] However, there was no system in place to ensure that he got treatment, and it's not clear whether he would have had access to adequate treatment had he been willing to go.

The high-profile tragedies have spurred rapid changes in the administrative response to determining risk. In the wake of Virginia Tech, many colleges and universities created "threat assessment teams," composed of counselors, faculty, deans, and sometimes lawyers. Virginia and Illinois actually passed laws mandating the establishment of such teams.[5] These are very important in attenuating risk, but they fall short of adequately addressing the larger problems of limited mental health care for students. In part, it's a resource allocation issue: universities are still figuring out how much it is within their scope of practice to also provide health services to their students. And in part, it's about recognizing that this population may have unique mental health needs, and that specialized training is necessary in providing optimal care.

After the public scrutiny that accompanies the media coverage of suicides or murders, some individual universities did increase funding to their counseling centers, expanding staffing and programming. But there's significant variability in mental health resources for students across institutions, for reasons including size of the institution, funding (public versus private), and geographic location. And psychiatric services in particular tend to be woefully inadequate. Psychiatrists accounted for less than 5% of counseling center full-time-equivalent hours in 2011.[6]

Historically, college counseling centers arose to meet the normal developmental and vocational needs of students, rather than their clinical needs. They focused on advising, counseling, and testing. As early as the 1950s, however, especially as soldiers returned to school after World War II, there was recognition of the growing need to provide comprehensive mental health services on college campuses in order to fully support the educational mission of institutions of higher learning. Influenced by the goals of the community mental health movement, which sought to integrate mental well-being into existing communities, Dana Farnsworth, M.D., articulated the psychiatrist's role on campus as both educational / consultative, collaborating with others to provide psychological support and preventive services, and clinical: taking care of those students who needed treatment.[7] But there's been uneven application of those goals, and especially of psychiatric care, across university communities in the last 60 years. As our understanding of mental health and illness has changed, and more medications make their way onto college campuses, it's critical to have a fuller understanding of college student mental health needs. And since the passage of the "new GI bill," the Post-9/11 Veterans Educational Assistance Act of 2008, millions of service members who served in Iraq and Afghanistan may be entering college, bringing with them yet another set of unique mental health needs and a swell in numbers perhaps similar to that seen post–World War II.

Do the mental health issues college students face really differ from those of their age-matched peers who are not enrolled in college? According to the most comprehensive study, using results from the 2002 National Epidemiologic Study on Alcohol and Related Conditions, they do.[8] Most striking is that the overall rate of psychiatric disorders in the 18- to 24-year-old age bracket is high, with about half having had a psychiatric disorder in the past year. Although the overall rate was not different for those attending college, alcohol use disorders were significantly more frequent among college students. Some problems, such as personality disorders and bipolar disorder, were lower among college students. Particularly disturbing was that college students were less likely to receive treatment for alcohol or drug addictions than their non-college-attending peers. Even with the upsurge in numbers at college counseling centers, most students who are identified as potentially depressed and even suicidal in surveys are not engaged in treatment.

The majority of college student mental health difficulties never end up in the public eye, yet they affect students' everyday lives in profound ways. When asked about the top 10 impediments to academic performance, students cited "stress" as number one, followed closely by "sleep difficulties, Internet use/computer games, depression/anxiety disorder/SAD," and "alcohol."[9] Most students reported feeling "overwhelmed" at least once during the past academic year, and nearly half felt "so depressed it was difficult to function" at least once; almost 1 in 10 "seriously considered suicide."[10] More and more students take psychotropic medications. Among students seen at college counseling centers, 24% now take medicine, compared with 9% in 1994.[11] This is likely an underestimate, since it doesn't include the students who receive therapy at the center but psychiatric medications from their family doctor, the campus student health center, or community psychiatrists. It also doesn't capture the students who never receive care at the counseling center but are in treatment in other settings.

In addition to causing academic underperformance, psychological problems have a range of other insidious effects, from creating difficulties in establishing friendships and other intimate relationships, to causing housing conflicts, delaying graduation, and contributing to dropping out of school. Depression can significantly influence whether a student remains in college.[12] And since universities are communities with various administrative systems in place, they provide enormous opportunities to intervene early in the course of a psychiatric illness and to alter the trajectory not only of the illness but also of the student's life.

CHAPTER 2

The Changing Face of the American University Student

Along with the general increase in the numbers of young adults attending college, the demographics of the students in American universities have been changing in the past few decades. To most effectively help students with their mental health concerns, it's essential to understand some of these changes and to be aware of the rapid pace of continued change that now seems to be the norm. College enrollment is increasing at a faster rate than in previous decades. Between 1997 and 2007 the numbers of registered students increased by 26%, compared with a 14% increase in the previous decade.[1] And the numbers are growing more rapidly for full-time than for part-time students.

Other interesting trends have emerged. Until around 1980, more men than women attended college, and then the ratio flipped. Women are now significantly overrepresented among undergraduates. This holds true, though the difference is smaller, for graduate school students as well. Since more women than men tend to present for mental health treatment, this may be one factor driving up the demand for campus mental health services.

Students from racial and ethnic groups traditionally in the minority make up more and more of the student body. Thirty-six percent of enrolled students identified as minorities in 2010, compared with 15% in 1976.[2] The most dramatic growth has been among young adults from Hispanic or Asian backgrounds, though there has also been an increase in the numbers of African American students. Minority students represent a much larger proportion of community college attendees, however, than they do of four-year public or private colleges. High school seniors from poorer families have significantly lower expectations of earning a bachelor's degree than do their wealthier peers.[3] Data on socioeconomic trends among students in four-year colleges over the past decade are hard to come by, but there is some evidence of increasing stratification based on income levels between more selective and less selective institutions, and between four-year and two-year colleges. Some of the most selective institutions have more generous financial aid packages, which might enable more academically qualified students from lower socioeconomic groups to attend. Students who struggle financially, however, or who come from families in lower socioeconomic groups, screen positive for depression and anxiety more frequently than do financially comfortable students,[4] so it's important to assess financial stressors in the course of evaluating students for mental health concerns.

Race, ethnicity, gender, and socioeconomic status can interact in complex, variable, and sometimes unpredictable ways, both in terms of university enrollment and with regard to progress and success in the university setting. A full discussion of this is beyond the scope of this chapter. The broad labels above clearly don't sufficiently capture the many cultures by which students define themselves. For example, students completing the NASPA Profile of Today's College Student survey were given the opportunity, if they were among the 8.3% who marked "Asian/Pacific Islander" as their race, to further specify "American" or a number of Asian ethnicities, such as "Bangladeshi," "Cambodian," "Chinese," and so on, more precisely pinpointing their background. In 2008, the most common response on that item was Chinese, (32%) followed by Filipino (17%), Vietnamese (15%), Indian (13%), and many other categories.[5] More students now identify as "biracial" or "multiracial."

More students are out about being gay, lesbian, bisexual, or transgender, but the majority are still not out to everyone, according to the 2008 NASPA Profile of Today's College Student. In the 1980s, the average age for beginning the coming out process was between 19 and 23; by 2011 the average age dropped to 16.[6] Even as college admissions officers tout the value of diversity and inclusiveness, however, and even as students themselves become more accepting of differences, students from underrepresented groups continue to face more challenges than their peers. With the advent of social media such as Facebook, along with the potential for students from underrepresented groups to find community and support, there are unfortunately also new forums in which students experience bullying or discrimination. This all affects mental health.

Some evidence shows that students from traditionally underrepresented ethnic groups use counseling services differently and present with slightly different symptoms or symptom severity when they do come in. This parallels findings in community utilization rates. In a large study of counseling utilization across 40 different universities, Caucasian students attended the greatest number of sessions, and Latino students the fewest.[7] African American and Asian students also attended fewer sessions than their Caucasian classmates, and Asian students reported the highest degree of distress at intake. Caucasian students had lower distress both at intake and at termination. All groups seemed to benefit about equally from treatment, as measured by scores on the OQ-45 questionnaire. Cultural background clearly affects a student's attitudes toward mental health problems and seeking help, but not the likelihood that treatment will be helpful. Those of us who care about student mental health must continually improve our multicultural skills if we are to be effective in reaching the greatest number of students in distress.

The importance of cultural sensitivity and of familiarity with cross-cultural psychiatry extends beyond working with American minority students. The American college campus is becoming more and more international, reflecting the globalization sweeping across our world. High school seniors in the United States complain about the growing difficulty of admission into selective colleges, and they're not imagining it. They have to compete not only against greater numbers of their American peers, but also against an expanding international student pool. In the last twenty years, international student enrollment has grown by over 62%.[8] The bulk of international students in the United States currently comes from Asia—China, Korea, India, and Japan[9]—but that is rapidly changing.

Universities are increasingly recruiting abroad. Remaining flexible and competitive in a global community is one incentive, but financial gain is another. Higher education is seen as one of the United States' most valuable exports: the Department of Commerce is now partnering with schools to help promote this "product" abroad.[10] There's been controversy over the practice of using "agents": recruiters who are local to the targeted country and who receive commissions based on the number of students they successfully deliver to an institution.[11] Considering this practice from the perspective of student mental health, it's hard to ignore the potential pitfall that some students might be brought to a campus for which they are not a good fit, or at least without adequate preparation for the many challenges of living not only in a new national culture, but in the American campus subculture.

International students face many unique issues that can affect their emotional well-being. In addition to the obvious challenges of acculturation, there's the inescapable link between visa status and student status. International students can't drop courses or take a semester off if it affects their full-time student status, because this would jeopardize their ability to remain in the United States. Likewise, becoming ill for any reason might threaten enrollment status—and necessitate a return to their home country, often cloaked in shame.

There are limited data on how international students differ from American students in their mental health concerns and use of counseling. Several studies suggest that both between-group and within-group differences merit attention and more careful delineation. (For more on international student issues, see chapter 10.)

Another change on college campuses in the last two decades has been the increase in older students. Today, more than 40% of university students are over age 25, including 35% of undergraduate students; the total number is predicted to grow to more than 8 million by 2016.[12] These students may have different mental health needs than their younger counterparts, but they're subject to the same campus cultural pressures, which often brings out similar issues and problems. At times, the experience of being a university student trumps other, more mature aspects of that person's life.

As disability laws have required accommodations for students with disabilities in high school, more of these students are able to go on to college. The number of college students with disabilities has doubled in the past couple of decades,[13] and yet the responsibility for advocating for services or accommodations shifts from the institution to the individual in college. Students whose parents or teachers helped coordinate services for them may often find themselves having to navigate institutional systems for themselves, even as they long to fit into a new environment without drawing attention to their differences. This places an additional developmental demand on these students, during a time when they are dealing with the same academic and social adjustments as their peers. Students with physical limitations may daily face campuses that are not entirely accessible, but they may also need extra help adapting psychologically to the constraints and challenges of the university environment.

The Post-9/11 Veterans Educational Assistance Act of 2008 has created yet another change in the face of the American college student, since this funding will allow about 2 million military members to begin or resume higher education pursuits. Students who are veterans of the most recent wars may experience unique challenges in the transition to college life. The Department of Veteran Affairs launched an online resource in 2009, specifically designed for university counseling personnel, providing training modules in PTSD, alcohol abuse, suicide prevention, and other mental health issues in student veterans, to help expand expertise in treating this special population.[14] In addition to the veterans themselves, we are now seeing more students affected by the prolonged wars because they have boyfriends, girlfriends, spouses, or parents serving in the military.

The ever-expanding diversity across multiple areas among university students poses challenges to psychiatrists even in defining what constitutes a "normal" developmental trajectory. We have to constantly update our knowledge base to stay current with new information about new populations while applying psychological theories and psychiatric and pharmacological understanding that does help explain human behavior across cultures. Perhaps most important, we have to remain curious, open, and flexible in our attitude toward our patients in order to form meaningful therapeutic alliances that will allow us to best help them.

CHAPTER 3

Generational Issues on Campus

The psychiatry resident is frustrated. He's treated Ellen, a 20-year-old Caucasian sophomore with depression, for the first three months of her spring semester. With antidepressant medication and therapy, Ellen has steadily improved, and she's pulled up her grades in all but one class: organic chemistry. She considered dropping the class to avoid a blemish on her transcript but decided to forge ahead. Now, as finals approach, the resident has received several voice messages from Ellen's father, increasingly concerned that if Ellen receives a bad grade it will affect her chances to get into medical school. Ellen would like to take the final exam but reserve the right to get a medical withdrawal if she does poorly. Her parents "don't want her to be penalized for having been depressed" and are encouraging her to talk to her dean and "be proactive." They'd also like to speak to the resident's supervisor to make sure "we're exploring all options." "Students today are so entitled," the resident complains. "And I get now what they mean by helicopter parents. I mean, she was depressed, but now she's not. Why would they think she should get special treatment? Maybe she just isn't good at organic chemistry."

Over-involved parents? Entitled students? Frustrated faculty?

Much of the developmental framework we are taught as psychiatrists focuses on the individual. But students enter the university community in cohorts, and understanding the historic forces and cultural events that shape specific generations enhances our ability to work with students, their families, and even our colleagues within the university community. The generational framework is based mostly on qualitative research, but there are a few quantitative studies as well. Although no generalizing descriptions will apply to every person, understanding generational groups is useful. Most students on campus today are part of the millennial generation, or Gen Y, while most faculty, including campus psychiatrists, belong to either the baby boomer generation or Gen X. Here's a brief overview of the different generations and ways in which their group characteristics might play out when we're working with students' psychiatric concerns.

The Millennial Generation (born 1981–2004)

Also called "Generation Me," the group comprising the majority of university students has been characterized as the most wanted group of children in history.[1] The most extensive descriptions come from the work of Neil Howe and William Strauss, authors of *Millennials Rising, Millennials Go to College,* and other research on generational differences. Howe and Strauss summarized their findings in seven words that have since influenced many people working with young adults, from university administrators to marketing executives to bosses in the workforce. According to Howe and Strauss, this generation is "special, sheltered, confident, team-oriented, achieving, pressured and conventional." It is also the largest generational cohort to date.

Every milestone in their lives has been a source of celebration. They've been protected, coming of age in an era of unprecedented safety consciousness among parents: the time of car seats, bicycle helmet laws, and school lockdowns. They're confident and goal oriented. Some studies have found higher rates of self-esteem, along with higher rates of narcissism, in this group. By the mid-1990s, the average college man had higher self-esteem than 86% of college men in 1968, with similar differences among college women.[2] This high self-esteem often leads to heightened expectations of themselves and of their institutions. Some studies suggest that an increase in narcissism leads students to believe they have a range of talents and abilities, making it harder to choose a career or even a major in college. Howe and Strauss's work, however, suggests that these kids have been on career tracks since elementary school.

Millennials tend to be more group oriented, not wanting to stand out among their peers.[3] They prefer egalitarian rather than hierarchical leadership. They are achievement oriented and often see college as a path to material success rather than a means of personal development. According to the 2011 American Freshman National Norms survey, getting a better job is the number one reason students cite for attending college these days.[4] This focus is often accompanied by a sense of pressure to succeed. Because millennials have had such highly structured, supervised lives, they may have difficulty with the decreased external structure of college, and especially graduate school. They may take on too many activities, and then expect others to be flexible with them in negotiating conflicts. They've been brought up to take advantage of every opportunity, so it may be difficult for them to withdraw from classes or activities, as it was for Ellen, the resident's patient.

Gen Y is also considered more conventional than previous generations, more likely to follow or establish social norms, and more in line with their parents' values than were previous generations.[5] Millennials have grown up with technology: they don't remember a time before computers, e-mail, or cell phones. They are "digital natives." They communicate more frequently with their parents, whose opinions they value, than did previous groups of college students. It's not unusual for students to be in daily contact with their families. This challenges the classical concepts of separation-individuation that many mental health professionals learned a generation ago, but again, understanding the culture helps prevent over-pathologizing behavior that may now be the norm.

College students in the new millennium tend to attribute the cause or control of events or outcomes to their environment or other factors outside themselves: they are more likely to believe in an external locus of control.[6] This may make them seem more passive, as they may blame factors outside themselves when things go wrong.

Some criticize these descriptions of the millennial generation as being too narrow, and especially bound by race, ethnicity, or socioeconomic status. Fred Bonner, a professor at Texas A&M University, argues that many minority college students might not recognize themselves in generational descriptions that include "special, sheltered, confident."[7] This is especially significant in the United States because this cohort is the most ethnically and culturally diverse group in history. An alternate model of the experience of African American millennials, also dubbed "Black Gen M," suggests that these young adults did not all grow up in economically stable conditions, nor do all feel protected by the government, indulged by their parents, or sheltered from the harsh realities of life.[8] This model encourages mindfulness to the heterogeneity of minority students. Bonner notes that for academically gifted black males, for example, the pressure to succeed that white millennials also experience may manifest itself as a perceived need to "be less black," leading to a loss of confidence.

Others question the findings on grounds of methodology. For example, Twenge and Campbell's findings that narcissistic traits were up in Gen Y held true in data from 27 campuses nationwide—but not in data from University of California, which is 40% Asian.[9] Twenge and colleagues speculated that this was because Asian cultures discourage narcissism, suggesting that Asian American students also may not fit as neatly into the white-culture American millennial-generation template. However, Trzesniewski and colleagues (who reported the University of California data) didn't find, in their studies, that Gen Y youth in general showed many cohort-related differences from the previous generation. They challenged the methodology of Twenge's studies as using small convenience samples rather than large mass-testing samples.

Although the traditional millennial lens may not fit every college student, its descriptors are prevalent on college campuses, and understanding it helps us understand the discussions that arise in our culture regarding generations. It thus can be a helpful starting point in placing students within a historical and cultural context.

Generation X (born 1961–1981)

This group, to which some older students on campus belong, and which will increasingly encompass parents of students, got a fair amount of media coverage in the 1990s as being the different younger generation—not unlike the current focus on the millennials. Gen X followed the baby boomers and is sometimes called the "baby buster" or "lost" generation. Many grew up as latchkey kids, because both the divorce rate and the percentage of children born outside of marriage doubled between 1965 and 1977,[10] and women entered the workforce in higher numbers. Although Gen X'ers are seen as more diverse and complex than previous generations, they are also less confident about the stability of jobs, earnings, and relationships. They married later and tended to live with their parents more often and for longer. They were the first generation to seem to delay entry into adulthood.

Generation X'ers have also been described as more cynical and pessimistic, with little confidence in social institutions and a tendency to be resourceful and independent.[11] They came of age in a time of rising crime and falling SAT scores, as well as the increasing threat of AIDS. They are considered to be risk takers in the workplace. They entered college in higher numbers than previous generations, but graduation rates didn't correspondingly rise, and incomes went down.[12]

Gen X parents are even more intensely involved in their children's lives than were boomer parents.[13] On average they communicate with their child nearly twelve times a week, and 70% have some input into their college student's course selection. They expect transparency from the colleges their children attend regarding grades, health records, and other information. Children of Gen X parents feel an even greater pressure to succeed and tend to expect their parents to intervene on their behalf when they encounter problems. Thus Ellen, in the vignette above, may have welcomed and encouraged her father's intervention in her academics and mental health care.

Baby Boomer Generation (born 1943–1960, or through 1964)

Baby boomers—children born into postwar prosperity—were the largest generation of their time. Their childhood homes were largely traditional and conformist, but they came of age during the sexual revolution and the consciousness-raising protests that encouraged placing value on individualism.[14] Baby boomers were indulged. Dr. Spock's work was influential on this cohort, emphasizing permissive parenting and a focus on creativity and curiosity. As a result, boomers, the best-educated generation to enter the workforce, tend to question authority and to seek meaningful work.[15] They believe in paying their dues, however, and some have stayed in lifelong jobs within a company. They tend to be involved in the world around them, fighting oppression. Their historical landmarks include the Vietnam War, the Civil Rights Movement, and the Kennedy and King assassinations. Boomers care less than other generations about what others think of them—even some quantitative data support this impression. Beginning in the 1950s, until the late 1970s, college students showed sharp decreases in their need for social approval, and this stabilized in the 1980s at a historically low level.[16]

As parents, baby boomers have been much more involved in raising their children than generations that preceded them. They were the first soccer moms and helicopter parents. The latter is especially relevant for work with current college students: these parents are accustomed to being involved in every moment of their children's lives, and for some of their children, the expectation is mutual. One study found that 40% to 60% of parents from all socioeconomic backgrounds can be classified as helicopter parents, and universities are increasingly offering parents avenues for constructive involvement in their children's lives.[17]

The Concept of Emerging Adulthood

Some who study generational trends have suggested that the boomers and the millennials have more similarities than differences. Certainly one common trait, seen in all of the last three generations, is a progressively delayed entry into what was traditionally seen as adulthood. Although this might be due to different dynamics—boomers rebelled against their parents' social timetable, while millennials are close to their parents and may delay work or moving out because they're trying to get everything just right—the trend seems to be continuing. Psychologist Jeffrey Arnett has conceptualized this as a new psychological developmental stage, which he calls "emerging adulthood," and which his research suggests is distinct from both adolescence and adulthood.

Emerging adulthood spans the ages 18 to 25 and is an in-between period, with significant identity exploration and focus on the self and on possibility. It is culture bound, occurring only in industrialized societies.[18] Post-industrial economies, which require higher educational levels for success, delay entry into the workforce. According to Arnett, two other historical forces have fueled the emergence of this stage: the increase in educational and work opportunities for women, and the sexual revolution, which uncoupled sex from marriage.

Emerging adults as a group are much more heterogeneous than either adolescents or adults. The late teens / early twenties age group experiences the greatest number of transitions, including the highest level of residential mobility. For many college students, their residential status changes every year, and often more than once a year (taking into account summer and other breaks, or semesters or a year abroad.)

Although adolescence is traditionally considered the developmental stage for identity formation, Arnett argues that identity is now consolidated in emerging adulthood. The explorations of adolescence are more tentative and transient, whereas by the late teens or early twenties, they're more focused and serious. Emerging adults date not only to have fun in the moment, but also as a way to move toward greater emotional and physical intimacy and to find a life partner. Similarly, they work not simply to obtain money for leisure but as a way to prepare for adult work roles. Not all the explorations of emerging adulthood are goal oriented, however; Arnett notes significant exploration for its own sake, especially of worldviews. College and graduate students, in particular, are exposed to worldviews that often differ from those of their families, and frequently they question views they've held, including religious and political beliefs. Even emerging adults who are not enrolled in higher education see defining their own beliefs and worldviews as necessary for attaining adult status.

Adolescence has also been commonly associated with risk-taking behaviors, but here again, Arnett's data suggest that certain risk-taking behaviors actually peak during emerging adulthood. These include binge drinking and other kinds of substance abuse, unprotected sex, driving while intoxicated, and speeding.[19] In part this may be due to the absence of specific defined roles for people during this time. For example, working adults have job responsibilities that limit when and how they may drink, and teens living at home likewise have curfews and parental supervision. But a college student who misses class because of a drinking binge may not be held accountable by anyone else, so problems may build before others notice.

The concept of continued risk taking during emerging adulthood is supported by new neurobiological findings about the continuing maturation of the human brain. The prefrontal cortex and other areas responsible for executive functioning and voluntary control of behavior show significant change into the early twenties. Although the basic tools of cognitive function are in place by adolescence, ongoing synaptic pruning and myelination, which occur after adolescence, allow consistent coordinated responses that rely on communication between multiple brain regions.[20] A recent MRI study of college freshmen found that within a six-month period in their first year, the greatest brain changes occur in the right midcingulate gyrus, inferior anterior cingulate gyrus, right caudate head, right posterior insula, and bilateral claustrum, all areas involved in integrating information and processing sensory input to arrive at appropriate behavioral responses.[21] Because the insula is involved in introception, these findings may demonstrate a biological basis for increasing self-awareness in college freshmen.

Our growing neurobiological understanding must influence our clinical responses to the psychopathology we encounter in emerging adults. Since the brain is still myelinating, interventions presented at later points in a college student's life may be more effective than when tried earlier, since that student's cognitive abilities may have solidified.

Perhaps as the brain continues to change, it is especially sensitive to certain kinds of experiences. According to psychologist Jennifer Tanner, not only is emerging adulthood a distinct developmental period in life, but it's also a critical juncture during which "marker events" are more strongly integrated into people's lives and memories than at other times in life.[22] The primary developmental task of young adulthood, she says, is "recentering," which Tanner conceptualizes as a three-stage process. First, adolescents transition into the emerging adult stage by shifting from the dependent roles of living with parents or other caretakers to relationships that are more mutual and reciprocal, requiring shared responsibility. Next is an experiential stage, during which they explore a series of possibilities in love, work, and worldview; commitments to roles and relationships tend to be transient. In the third stage, certain role commitments are solidified, as people move into marriage or partnerships, jobs, and sometimes parenthood. Goals shift from being focused on academics, friendship, and leisure to a focus on occupation, family, and health.

Many cognitive abilities peak during emerging adulthood, including general intelligence, numerical ability, verbal aptitude, clerical perception, and finger dexterity. Emerging adults are more sensitive to emotional stimuli than older people, especially to fear and other negative experiences.[23] This may be due to continued maturation of the medial prefrontal cortex, a brain region involved in integrating emotional processes with information derived from internal and external sources. The potential for personality change is also greatest during this period. This challenges us in our clinical work, to not be overzealous in diagnosing pathology. What may look like a personality disorder in an 18-year-old may actually be within the range of normal variability.

Although emerging adulthood does not exist as a stage across all cultures, the historical forces that led to it are spreading globally. It's prevalent across many different regions, including Europe, Latin America, and Asia. People across the world increasingly delay marriage and childbirth as more women seek education and enter the workforce. Tanner and Arnett acknowledge that socioeconomic forces may constrain the experience of emerging adulthood, but according to available data, there are few differences between working-class and middle-class emerging adults. Further research should clarify any differences with regard to race, ethnicity, or sexual orientation, but existing information supports emerging adulthood as a normative developmental stage in post-industrial countries and as a useful concept in working with university students.

CHAPTER 4

The Psychiatrist's Role in College Mental Health

As the nature of the college counseling center has changed over time, so too has the role of the psychiatrist in providing mental health care to university students. Yet at the same time, some of the challenges we face now are not that different from those our predecessors grappled with as they tried to define best models of care. A brief historical perspective can help ground our understanding of our roles as we move forward.

The mental hygiene movement, which swept college campuses at the beginning of the twentieth century, focused on preventing emotional problems through an emphasis on developmental and contextual factors,[1] in contrast to a more medical, pathology-oriented model. This not only separated counseling from student health, and at times from psychiatry or "mental health centers," but also sometimes led to tensions between these models of care. Some of these tensions persist today. Psychiatrists usually served limited roles within counseling centers or were housed at student health clinics. At many universities, they didn't have a role on campus at all but worked in the community surrounding the university and were available to students as needed. In more rural or impoverished parts of the country, this remains the model today, and access to psychiatric care for students is limited.

The community mental health (CMH) movement of the 1960s advocated for a more integrated model of care, uniting the mental hygiene ideals with new knowledge about the clinical care of psychiatric illness. Paul Barreira, a psychiatrist who now heads Harvard University's Health Services, has written and spoken at national psychiatric meetings about how the principles of CMH are particularly relevant to college mental health services. First, CMH principles posit that services be community based, for a well-defined population. Second, CMH models pay attention to general well-being, through prevention strategies and educational programming. Third, clinicians working within the system must be able to accurately and rapidly identify more serious emotional problems and appropriately refer for treatment. Last, the clinicians within the system must also be capable of providing evidence-based treatment that meets current standards of care. All these clearly apply in the care of university students, since the university represents a well-defined community. Barreira emphasizes that services must be culturally informed, must invite student participation, and must periodically undergo evaluation.

In the last decade there's been an increase in the numbers of psychiatrists working in college mental health. Groups such as the American Psychiatric Association and the National Network of Depression Centers have formed task forces to focus specifically on this topic. Fellowship programs in child and adolescent psychiatry are increasingly interested in including emerging adults within their scope of care. The role of psychiatrists in providing care to this population is growing.

The Psychiatrist on Campus

According to the 2011 National Survey of College Counseling Center Directors (NSCCCD), which represents 228 centers across the United States, 64% of centers have access to on-campus psychiatric consultation. Some of these psychiatrists work within counseling centers and some within student health clinics. The exact role of the psychiatrist depends somewhat on the location of his or her appointment and varies between institutions according to how well staffed the institution is. Many universities have only one on-campus psychiatrist, and that person may work only part time. That often limits their role to medication evaluation and management and crisis evaluation.

But psychiatrists, whose training emphasizes the bio-psycho-social aspects of emotional problems and mental illness, have much to offer college students—and the university community—beyond medication management. Although tight resource allocation may not allow many to practice much traditional psychotherapy—most campus psychiatrists do not have the time to carry a case-load of weekly, hour-long therapy cases even if working in a brief therapy model—the most effective psychiatric approach to working with students calls for a psychotherapeutic stance even within the 20- to 30-minute medication management visit. This is what often makes the difference in a student's decision to take or not take a particular medication, or to follow another recommended course of treatment.

> Twenty-three-year-old Li, a Chinese international first-year graduate student, is referred by the student health service physician for counseling and sees a therapist at the counseling center for intake. He's been experiencing fatigue, loss of motivation, and anxiety attacks, although Li objects to the last characterization, and he continues to believe a physical problem is causing his bouts of nervousness, tachycardia, and shortness of breath. The student health physician prescribed low-dose clonazepam, but the student has not taken any of the medication. The counselor recommends a brief course of cognitive behavioral therapy and explains the rationale. The student insists he has no time for this and is frustrated with having been referred to the counseling center at all for his medical problems. Exasperated, the counselor convinces him to meet with the psychiatrist for a second opinion about the clonazepam.

It's not uncommon for a student to have received an antidepressant or anti-anxiety medication prescription from a nonpsychiatric physician or nurse practitioner, only to refuse to fill the prescription. Treatment of depression and anxiety more often occurs within the primary care setting, both in the general population and among college students.[2] Simple recommendations about safe treatments may seem clear cut to us clinicians but to previously healthy emerging adults, they seem like life-altering, monumental choices, and in some senses, they are. To choose to take a medicine that in some ways alters the mind, when most university students value their minds and ability to think clearly perhaps above much else, is not a trivial decision. For students from certain countries, or from certain ethnic or religious backgrounds within the United States, additional cultural forces make the thought of psychiatric medication unacceptable and frightening. Psychiatrists working on campus need to understand all this and have the time to sensitively process it with their patients.

For most students, referral to a psychiatrist is a big deal: usually it is their first contact with this type of care. They come with preconceived fears and assumptions. An effective campus psychiatrist, therefore, must pass what one colleague calls the "curbside test." If the student were to run into the psychiatrist out on the street, would the psychiatrist stand out as odd, standoffish, or cold, or would he or she seem like a "real person"? Emerging adults fear the stereotypes they've seen in the movies: the quiet, analytic psychiatrist who asks questions and withholds explanations or information. In my experience students seem reassured when we are warm, take an active approach, avoid jargon, and don't talk down to them. They appreciate it when we have a good understanding of the specifics of their campus experience, from academic demands to administrative issues to the social life.

In working with a student like Li, we have to resist the impulse to insist that he either take medication or do cognitive behavioral therapy (or both). Our role is to recommend the best treatment options and then help Li make a decision. Of course, we could always say he "refused treatment" and move on to the next patient in line. But students like Li are suffering and often will engage in treatment that is effective for them if we just take a more patient, educational, collaborative stance. This may not be possible in all settings and is certainly not a hallmark of our mental health care system outside higher education. But within institutions of higher education, it seems to me that we can find a way to make health care an educational experience. Doesn't teaching students to take care of their mental and physical health allow them to then make the most of their college opportunities and, in this way, support the fundamental mission of universities? College mental health that aspires to this approach could become a model for effective mental health care in other settings too.

A study of depression treatment among a large national sample of college students found that only 22% received "minimally adequate" treatment, including both psychotherapy and psychopharmacology.[3] Among the group treated with medicine, however, 69% of those treated by a psychiatrist received minimally adequate care, compared with only 39% of those treated by a primary care provider. Rates for minority students, especially Asian students, were lower. This is an embarrassingly low bar: surely we can aim higher.

In cases like Li's, the psychiatrist's role might be more heavily educational, explaining the rationale behind labeling Li's symptoms as panic. Usually psychiatrists have more time for these discussions than do primary care providers. Psychoeducation might include reading materials about the risks and benefits of psychotropic medication or therapy. An SSRI antidepressant might be more helpful for Li's panic, but given his reluctance to even episodically take an as-needed benzodiazepine, he might balk even more at the suggestion of a daily antidepressant unless it's presented in the context of a good treatment alliance.

It's important to understand Li's ideas regarding what might help him and see whether we can fit our understanding of psychiatric symptom management into his framework. Sometimes a student's family member will have recommended another course of treatment; families of international students occasionally send traditional medications from home. With the student's permission, our educational role might extend to the family. If the student isn't in crisis and there are no significant risk factors for harm, we might first try the approaches the student proposes, even if they seem to have a low probability of success. We might know from experience that recurrent depression is unlikely to remit rapidly without treatment, but if a student insists that she wants to wait a few more weeks because she's felt better the past two days, then a helpful intervention might be to review symptoms to monitor, agree on a safety plan, and make a follow-up appointment in two weeks.

The psychiatrist on campus must sometimes be a case manager, helping students with a host of problems, from advocating for housing changes to consulting with professors, deans, advisers, or other campus professionals. At universities where a case manager position exists, enlisting that person's help is invaluable. Challenges arise from these multiple roles, however. It's important to be clear about when our role is entirely clinical, when consultative, and when there may be a conflict of interest between roles. Confidentiality remains paramount, but in some situations—when there's a high risk of danger to the student or to others in the university community—confidentiality is secondary to safety. In those cases the psychiatrist within a counseling or health center has the luxury of colleagues with whom to consult, and consulting is critically important.

Many university counseling centers are also training centers, usually for psychology or social work interns, but often also for psychiatry residents. The psychiatrist's role can then also include training. Sometimes psychiatrists directly supervise non-M.D. trainees in a one-to-one setting, but this is rare. More commonly they train informally, by modeling good interdisciplinary interactions, both in team settings and when they share cases. Psychiatrists who remain approachable to trainees and who help them understand the principles of how to refer appropriately for medication evaluation are serving both a training and a clinical function.

College counseling centers are excellent training sites for psychiatry residents, exposing them to greater diversity than they may have seen in other settings. Most students are also great candidates for psychotherapy. If supervising residents, the senior psychiatrist may need to develop a more formal didactic curriculum and take on a bigger training role, as well as one of coordinating with the resident's home institution and training director.

A challenge that arises for psychiatry residents and even for younger permanent psychiatrists working with college students is the possibility of overly identifying with the students. After all, we've had the college experience ourselves, and being back on campus can reactivate memories or attitudes. Residents in the same generational cohort as their patients may view the student's stressors and anxieties as normal and underdiagnose or undertreat. It's important to address this possibility in supervision. At the same time, judicious and appropriate self-disclosure can greatly help students. For example, helping an anxious pre-med student gain some perspective about grades by saying, "I had classmates who got a C and still got into medical school" or "yes, sitting in classes eight hours a day in medical school is hard, isn't it?" can be very helpful.

Mid-career psychiatrists are often in the same generation as the students' parents. This can cause issues with transference and counter-transference in the therapy—and even in medication management. Students may expect us to act like their parents and tell them what to do as well as resist if we are too directive. Sometimes in interactions with parents over the phone or in person, we may overly identify with *them*, and this can threaten our alliance with the student. In most cases, though, having permission to speak with parents is an invaluable opportunity to educate and to solicit their support of treatment. I've worked with many students over the years who were reluctant to take medicine because they believed their parents would be opposed to it, and the parents were opposed because they didn't understand the situation. When those parents were given a patient explanation of their child's condition and of the risks and benefits of treatment, their support of it helped the student accept and adhere to the treatment.

The Private Practice or Community Psychiatrist Serving Students

Even universities that have multiple on-campus psychiatrists are not able to meet all the psychiatric needs of their student populations without referring some students out for care. At schools without on-campus psychiatrists, the community psychiatrists are a vital resource. Psychiatrists who want to expand their work to incorporate college students can be most helpful if they keep in mind the importance of the developmental framework. They too must be prepared to work collaboratively, with the student and, at times, with parents, university faculty, or case managers. Ways to make a private practice more student-friendly include:

- Help students navigate the complexities of their medical insurance.
- Make some sliding-scale fees available, for students who are unable to afford full fee and lack adequate insurance.
- Remain sensitive to cross-cultural issues in psychiatry, and maintain an attitude of curiosity and humility toward students whose backgrounds and experience may differ widely from our own.
- Start medications at low doses and increase more slowly than usually done with adult patients.
- Have hours available that dovetail with student academic schedules. Students particularly love evening and weekend hours; early morning hours are much less popular.
- Be close to campus, or close to public transportation, if available.

PART II / CLINICAL CHALLENGES

CHAPTER 5

Sleep Problems on Campus

Dave is a 19-year-old biracial sophomore from Texas who is having persistent difficulty falling asleep. He has come to the counseling center psychiatrist via referral from one of the psychology interns. He had initially gone to the student health service. When zolpidem was ineffective but clonazepam helped, the student health doctor suggested there might be an anxiety component to his insomnia and referred him to the counseling center. Dave was frustrated about having to talk to a counselor, however, insisting he just needed sleeping pills.

Evaluating Symptoms: The Campus Context

The challenge in evaluating sleep disturbances in university students is that they are so common, they seem normal—even inevitable—to both students and faculty. Adolescent shifts in chronobiology cause a normal delay in both sleep onset and wake onset, meaning later to bed and later to rise is normal for teens. The campus culture accentuates this, sometimes to the degree that sleep cycles are reversed. The college lifestyle has never been conducive to good sleep, but in the twenty-first century, there are even more challenges. Students are sleeping fewer hours on average than a generation ago. According to the American College Health Association's 2009 National College Health

Assessment (NCHA),[1] sleep difficulties are second only to "stress" on a list of factors that students report have negatively affected their academic performance. Other studies suggest as many as a third of college students suffer from regular, severe sleep problems, and barely over a tenth meet criteria for good sleep quality.[2]

Sleep deprivation is not benign: it can lead to accidents, illness, and, of course, underachievement in school. Insomnia can also be a harbinger of the more serious psychiatric conditions that often first appear in the late teens and early twenties. A thorough and systematic evaluation through the lens of understanding campus culture is essential. All insomnia evaluations should start with an assessment of the most common barriers to sleep on today's campuses.

Students seeking professional help with sleep typically first approach a primary care doctor or their student health center, so that by the time a psychiatrist steps in, simple transient insomnia is a less likely diagnosis. It's still worthwhile to explicitly review the modifiable factors in the student's environment, especially those listed in table 5.1. It's also best practice to do a complete psychiatric evaluation, including a good history, full mental status examination, risk assessment, and some screening for common psychiatric problems.

In his intake appointment with the psychiatrist, Dave admits to using energy drinks to stay awake but notes that they're "natural, without caffeine." He reluctantly reports drinking alcohol about four nights per week, between three and eight drinks per occasion, but does not think this affects his sleep since on the nights he drinks, typically Thursday through Sunday, he has less trouble sleeping. His fraternity brothers drink just as much or more, he insists, but they seem unaffected by insomnia. Dave describes himself as biracial, with a Chinese-born father and Caucasian American mother, but when asked whether he experiences flushing or other physical effects when drinking, he bristles and says he tolerates alcohol just fine.

Dave often stays up until 1 a.m. on weeknights to finish schoolwork, and then typically can't fall asleep until 2 or 3. He has to wake at 8 for a morning class three days a week. On the weekends, he's often up until 4 a.m. socializing and sleeps in until noon or later to catch up.

Because of the high prevalence of alcohol and other substance use on campus, questions about frequency, amount, and consequences of alcohol and other drug use must be a part of every insomnia evaluation. At Duke we routinely gather this information as part of the intake paperwork, and then home in on

Table 5.1   Common contributors to sleep problems on campus

Erratic schedule; irregular bedtime
Stress (about school, worry about the future)
Room too bright, hot, cold, noisy, etc.
Alcohol use
Caffeine use, including energy drinks
Over-the-counter sleep aid use
Weight-loss drug use
Other drug use (particularly stimulants: student's own or diverted from others)
Electronics (computers, cell phones, etc.)
Video games

Source: Lund, H. G., Reider, B. D., & Whiting, A. B., et al. (2010). "Sleep Patterns and Predictors of Disturbed Sleep in a Large Population of College Students." *Journal of Adolescent Health, 46,* 124–32.

pertinent positive answers. Students sometimes become defensive or frustrated, thinking these questions don't relate to their primary complaint. The more patient and nonjudgmental we can be in our approach, the more likely it is that we will get honest information, which will allow more opportunities for effective intervention.

As health professionals, we know that there are differences in alcohol metabolism rates based on gender, weight, race, and other factors, but students often have a cursory understanding of these factors or dismiss them. In Dave's case, his Chinese ancestry is relevant, increasing the odds that he might have deficiencies in the alcohol-metabolizing enzymes, but for emerging adults, questions of culture and background can incite complex emotional reactions. If, for example, Dave's father is more authoritarian and prizes academic achievement, and Dave was an excellent student through high school but began to socialize more in college, turning away from some of his father's values, he may be reluctant to identify with anything he views as stereotypically Asian. If Dave doesn't have an enzyme deficiency and can biologically tolerate alcohol, cultural forces may still be contributing. For example, if he is a minority student within his fraternity, he might dive into the drinking culture as the most visible way to fit in. It's standard best practice for psychiatrists to establish a strong therapeutic alliance, provide accurate information, and float some hypotheses. In working with someone like Dave—smart, sleepless, drinking too much, and defensive with mental health care providers—the challenge is achieving this without making him feel patronized.

Students frequently overestimate the drinking and drug use behavior of their peers. According to the NCHA, almost 69% of students reported "any alcohol use" within the past 30 days, but they estimated that over 95% of their peers were drinking during that same period. Similarly, in this national sample of over 87,000 students, only 14% reported any other substance use (tobacco, marijuana, or other illegal drugs) in the previous month, but they estimated that 77% of their classmates had used in that same period. It's likely that they also misperceive how their peers' drinking behavior affects sleep and general function. Students are surprised and sometimes skeptical when confronted with this information, but it can be a powerful tool to help put their own substance use into perspective. Regardless of how their use compares to their peers', these conversations are an invaluable opportunity for us to educate students about the depressant effects of alcohol and some drugs, and about their actual effects on sleep. Information about the withdrawal effects on sleep of stimulants, both prescription and illegal, is likewise important. Though often reluctant to eliminate partying from their lifestyle in order to get a good night's sleep, many students will agree to a trial period of cutting back or eliminating substances.

A relatively new substance category on campus is the energy drink, introduced to the United States in 1997. Energy drink use has exploded in the past decade. Between 2002 and 2006, the U.S. energy drink market increased from $100 million to over $600 million, with little regulatory oversight and much aggressive marketing, to adolescent males in particular.[3] Drinks touted as being "natural" or even "decaf" often still contain caffeine, albeit in smaller doses. Many contain taurine, glucuronolactone, and choline; in combination these can have stimulant effects. Some contain guarana, a Brazilian berry with seeds richer in caffeine than coffee beans. Most energy drinks also contain high quantities of sugar. The limited research that exists suggests that energy drinks are popular on campus and increasing in popularity, with 34% of 18- to 24-year-olds regularly consuming them. Most students use them to stay alert to study, but as many as a quarter are combining energy drinks with alcohol in the belief that they'll feel less intoxicated, leading to a rise in alcohol-related negative consequences, such as sexual assault and injuries or illness requiring medical attention[4] (see chapter 6 on alcohol use). This is a new and concerning phenomenon on campus, with the highest reported rates among young males, athletes, and members of fraternity or sorority houses. And clearly, this combination can even more seriously disrupt sleep.

In the case above, Dave is hoping for a pill that will get him to sleep without having to sacrifice his sleep-interfering lifestyle habits. For the prescribing physician, the fact that Dave specifically requests a benzodiazepine poses several challenges. First, most of us have been trained to avoid potentially addictive medications in people with or recovering from an addiction. Second, even in the absence of addiction, Dave is clearly drinking too much alcohol and may have a higher tolerance to benzodiazepines. He has several unhealthy habits and the attitude that there is a substance for everything that ails him. How can a physician justify prescribing something that may help with insomnia but will perpetuate an unhealthy lifestyle? And finally, what if there is an underlying mood or anxiety disorder? A benzodiazepine in that case would really be a Band-aid rather than an accurate treatment.

There is no treatment model that will work in every case, of course, but in general I've found that prioritizing the treatment alliance early on, and then taking a longer-term view of treatment goals, can be invaluable. We're all living in a culture of instant gratification, and not only does the student want his problem fixed immediately, but we often feel pressure to treat efficiently and move on. Many campus counseling centers have session limits, putting obstacles in the way of a longitudinal treatment model. Yet today's campus generation has been bombarded with so much advertising—as well as with health information—that they're used to tuning out. They don't always distinguish between accurate information and its opposite, and they need help sorting through the barrage of data in ways that promote health. Information in the context of an authentic relationship is harder to ignore, but it takes time to build an authentic relationship.

How does this relate to the question of prescribing benzodiazepines for insomnia? In most cases, they are not the first treatment approach we'd use (see below for more on alternatives). But when significant anxiety is triggering insomnia, or when a student has had a good response to a benzodiazepine and specifically asks for one, very cautious, limited use can be therapeutic. Students who are not suffering from addiction understand which substances are risky and prefer to avoid them; most use prescribed benzodiazepines with caution and as prescribed. In Dave's case, it's helpful to lay out the risks and benefits of benzodiazepine use as well as of alcohol and energy drinks, to engage him in an experiment in which he'll gradually cut back on and even eliminate the latter two, and to do a thorough review of sleep hygiene. Within this framework, judicious short-term use of a low-dose benzodiazepine can be helpful. If I were to give a prescription for clonazepam to Dave, I'd prescribe 0.5mg at bedtime and supply only ten tablets, with no refills. If I have concerns that he might already be addicted and doctor shopping or pill seeking, I can check with pharmacy registries to see if he has obtained other controlled substances from other providers. But in my clinical experience and that of my colleagues, students with a presentation like Dave's, after careful screening to rule out addiction, can get significant relief from brief benzodiazepine use.

Recent British Association for Psychopharmacology guidelines recommend short-acting benzodiazepines when using this class for insomnia,[5] but a longer-acting benzodiazepine such as clonazepam may have less potential for addiction. In addition to providing symptom relief, restoring sleep is a critical risk-reduction strategy: insomnia is a risk factor for both suicide and violence. All these factors must be weighed in the judicious use of benzodiazepines.

For someone with Dave's presentation, a benzodiazepine cannot, of course, constitute the entire treatment. It buys time, providing further opportunities to emphasize good sleep habits and teach nonpharmacologic approaches to healthy sleep. Students underestimate the havoc caused by irregular schedules. It's common for them to sleep deprive themselves during the week to meet academic demands and assume they'll catch up on sleep on the weekends. However, it takes longer than a day or two to physiologically make up for lost sleep, and the strategy of delaying wake times on the weekend perpetuates or exacerbates their insomnia. Teaching sleep hygiene improves sleep, especially when we emphasize consistently regular rise times.[6] Interesting new research done at Duke also suggests that social rhythms affect sleep among undergraduates: regular social engagement, particularly at earlier times of the day, improves sleep.[7] Exercise in the early part of the day helps too.

At our counseling center we've developed brochures that describe good sleep hygiene practices, and we distribute these along with sleep logs to help students make the connections. Students document not only hours slept, daytime sleep, and daytime wakefulness, but also drug and alcohol use and exercise. A focus on regular sleep schedules in conjunction with increased exercise and decreased alcohol and other substance use, within the context of a supportive treatment relationship, often clears up sleep problems and teaches students good health habits for life.

Sometimes students dismiss the focus on sleep hygiene because they're convinced it's "stress" that is interfering with their sleep, and they feel helpless to change the sources of their stress. They commonly describe being kept awake by ruminative worries about grades, jobs, or social situations. In the NCHA,

42% of students reported "more than average stress" in the past 12 months, and nearly 10% reported "tremendous stress." Although a subset of these students may be experiencing an anxiety or mood disorder, for others this is part of the normal developmental process of adjusting to college—and learning how to handle stress in healthy ways. Many college counseling centers offer groups or workshops that teach stress-management techniques. Cognitive behavioral therapies developed specifically for insomnia are a very effective treatment. In fact, guidelines for insomnia treatment recently released by the British Association for Psychopharmacology recommended CBT-i as a first-line treatment.[8] CBT-i is a manualized, multimodal approach that includes sleep restriction, stimulus-control, and cognitive restructuring.

Emerging adults respond well to cognitive behavioral therapies in general. There aren't many studies examining insomnia treatment techniques specifically in university students, but at least one recent study suggested that students with sleep difficulties can learn to "worry constructively," leading to improved sleep.[9] Students are instructed to write down, during an early evening time block (6 to 8 p.m.), at least three worries that have been keeping them up and the first steps toward a solution. They then fold their list in half and keep it near their bed, and if worry crops up as they try to fall asleep, they remind themselves they have already done what they can to deal with the worry.

Another strategy to help students deal with developmental stress is to teach them mindfulness meditation. Psychiatrists Holly Rogers and Margaret Maytan created a mindfulness meditation program specifically tailored for university students and described in detail in their book *Mindfulness for the Next Generation.* At Duke they run several mindfulness meditation groups each year, and we also provide individual students with mindfulness meditation exercises on CD or via online files, which they can download onto their computer or MP3 player and practice on their own. Meditation has many stress-relieving properties that last throughout the day. There's good evidence that combining mindfulness meditation with cognitive behavioral techniques is effective in treating insomnia.[10] Though this has not been tested specifically in college students, participants in the meditation program at Duke report improved sleep,[11] and there's growing evidence from other sources as well.

Although Dave did not find zolpidem helpful, many students with insomnia do get significant relief from short-term use of a sedative-hypnotic medicine. The British Association for Psychopharmacology has found the best evidence for the "z-drugs," such as zolpidem, zaleplon, and eszopiclone.

When Insomnia Is Associated with a Psychiatric Diagnosis

At his initial appointment, Dave agrees to cut back on alcohol and to eliminate energy drinks and daytime naps, in return for a limited (10-day, low-dose) prescription of clonazepam. He misses his two-week follow-up appointment but returns a month later, having run out of the medication and requesting more. Dave reports success in cutting back on drinking, which proved to him, he says, that he does not in fact have a problem with alcohol. When he's not drinking, however, he has a hard time at parties, feeling self-conscious and even panicky on occasion. He had to leave a party on the pretext of having a migraine when he felt flushed, short of breath, and like girls were sniggering about him. He thinks no one wants to hang out with him when he's not drinking, because he's much less interesting than his peers. His physical appearance bothers him, his small stature compared to his fraternity brothers, and he worries about his attractiveness. He admits to shyness in high school that was mitigated by the respect he got for being the smartest kid in his grade, and also by getting to know all his classmates within his small private school. In the past week, he's resumed drinking, because "it's not worth it to be in college and stressing all the time."

When students feel heard and trust their physician, even those who are wary of counselors may reveal symptoms that did not emerge in the initial evaluations. In the vignette above are several red flags for a social anxiety disorder diagnosis. As many as half of patients with a diagnosis of insomnia ultimately also have a psychiatric diagnosis.[12] (See figure 5.1 and table 5.2.) While asking further directed questions to see whether he fulfills DSM criteria for social anxiety, I'd remain mindful of the issues unique to college students. Remembering Arnett's principles of emerging adulthood (as discussed in chapter 3), I'd consider his complaints within the cultural norms of the student body at his particular university. In my case, working at an elite selective private college, I frequently encounter students for whom starting college is a narcissistic injury—a sense of self-efficacy is lost as their previous assumptions about themselves and the world are challenged. At Duke, with recent acceptance rates of less than one in nine, someone who is temperamentally shy, or who concentrated all his energy on academic success in order to build a competitive application for college—at the expense, perhaps, of developing social skills—might look as if he has social anxiety disorder as he transitions to the competitive college environment (see chapter 14 on anxiety and chapter 9 on perfectionism).

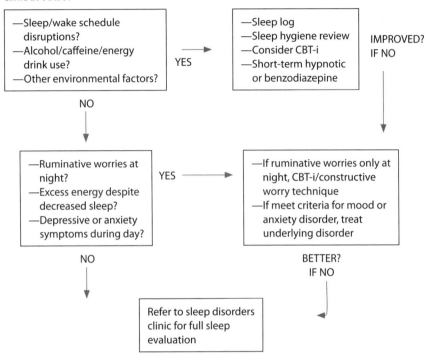

Figure 5.1. Algorithm for Evaluating Insomnia on Campus.

This may seem less likely in someone who is not a first-year student, but it's always worth asking about recent transitions. Each year of college brings significant changes for most students. Dave, a sophomore, may have just started living in a fraternity house and may be new to juggling the social demands of Greek life with academic demands. Other subgroups of students also face new social milieus that can cause difficulties. International students, for example, sometimes experience significant social anxiety that they claim they did not notice in their home country, as do students from underrepresented racial or ethnic groups and first-generation college students. Sometimes supporting a student's adjustment as he grapples with issues of identity and belonging, and helping him advocate for himself if there are issues of oppression, can make all

Table 5.2   Psychiatric conditions that present
with sleep disturbance

Major depressive disorder
Bipolar disorder
Generalized anxiety disorder
Obsessive compulsive disorder
Panic disorder
Post-traumatic stress disorder
Schizophrenia and other psychotic disorders

the difference in reducing what at first may appear to be symptoms of psychopathology. If functioning is sufficiently impaired, though, a trial of a serotonin-reuptake inhibitor can facilitate even this process. Often, group therapy is enormously helpful, though the students who most need it are the most reluctant to try it.

If I'm considering a social anxiety diagnosis, I'd also want to rule out other anxiety disorders. Although this would have been done at the initial evaluation, I'd revisit those questions now that the student reports emergence of symptoms after several weeks of sobriety. Positive family history and positive personal past history of psychiatric problems would sway me toward a psychiatric diagnosis. As with any patient, I'd take a collaborative, informative approach in recommending treatment: usually medication management combined with therapy. But university students sometimes respond differently to the suggestion to take antidepressants.

For example, Dave—despite using liberal amounts of alcohol, energy drinks, sleep aids, and perhaps other drugs—may be reluctant to take a medication that "messes with" his brain. It's important to understand what Dave is afraid of, and what kinds of stigma he might attach to the idea of taking a "brain-altering" medicine. Students in college are rightfully proud of their intellectual abilities and need reassurance that antidepressants won't dull their minds. Relying on our treatment relationship, correcting misconceptions, and taking a firm but gentle stance will increase the odds that Dave will adhere to the recommended treatment.

Although awakening too early—terminal insomnia—is more commonly associated with depression, in college students we see the full spectrum of sleep difficulties with mood disorders. Some, with hypersomnia, are referred to us once the health center has eliminated other possible causes of persistent fatigue. Often, treating the underlying mood or anxiety disorder relieves the sleep difficulty.

Sometimes treating a student with an antidepressant improves mood, anxiety, and concentration, but not the sleep complaint. Because some antidepressants exacerbate insomnia, if a sleep problem arises or persists during antidepressant treatment, switching medicines may become necessary. If daytime fatigue is significant and continues in the absence of other possible etiologies (such as a viral illness, thyroid problems, or anemia) or if the student admits to snoring or any symptoms of narcolepsy, it's good practice to refer him for a sleep study. Sometimes obstructive sleep apnea is the culprit. Frequently, however, sleep study results come back normal. If the difficulty falling asleep persists, I choose a more sedating antidepressant. I don't generally start with the sedating antidepressants because once the depression and insomnia improve, most students don't tolerate the concomitant weight gain and sedation that can persist with these agents.

Of course, if significant insomnia emerges during treatment with an antidepressant, I'd do a careful rescreening for the possibility of treatment-emergent mania or a bipolar disorder that hadn't been revealed in the original history.

Unless beginning treatment with a sedating antidepressant, it's important to simultaneously treat the insomnia that was a presenting complaint. Short-term use of a sedative-hypnotic during the first few weeks of antidepressant titration is often helpful; again, the "z-drugs" (zolpidem, zaleplon, eszopiclone) or the short-acting benzodiazepines, which all work on the GABA-A receptor, are good first-line treatments.

It's helpful to be patient with students who have a complex presentation and an attitude to treatment like Dave's. Although it can seem as if they're trying to manipulate the physician or refuse appropriate treatment (antidepressant in this case) while demanding a drug with abuse potential (clonazepam), they often *do* take in what we're telling them—it just may take longer. I've treated several students similar to Dave who refused treatment as freshmen or sophomores, or who dropped out of treatment when I refused to provide ongoing benzodiazepines as their substance use persisted, only to return to treatment later in the course of their time in college, making significant progress by their junior or senior years. I take their concerns seriously even when they minimize them or are dismissive, and I try to maintain a matter-of-fact, nonpreachy style while repeatedly stressing the points I consider most relevant to their successful treatment. Of course, the luxury of waiting is only an option when there are no risk factors for imminent danger.

When Day and Night Reverse

What about the students who practice good sleep hygiene, eliminate alcohol and caffeine, and still can't fall asleep? It's important to clarify how many hours of daytime sleep they are getting.

Some students stay up very late and then can't get up for class or other activities, or when forced to get up are so sleepy they can't fully participate in campus life. This may be a combination of genetic factors (some of us are wired to be more awake in the evenings than the mornings) and a phase delay in the circadian rhythms that govern sleep. This delay is similar to jetlag, but more persistent and impairing. Called delayed sleep phase syndrome and considered a circadian rhythm sleep-wake disorder in the DSM, this diagnosis is more common in young adults than in the rest of the population. A recent study of 191 students at a large, rural American university found that 11.5% qualified for this diagnosis, nearly double the rate in the general population.[13]

For some students, difficulty falling asleep persists until they're drifting off in the early morning hours and sleeping during the day. This pattern becomes engrained and differs from typical insomnia because these students are actually getting sufficient sleep; they are just out of sync with the usual day and night schedule of everyone else on campus. Anecdotally, it seems to be more common in graduate students who, untethered from class schedules, keep increasingly irregular hours. This seems to be an extreme form of delayed sleep phase syndrome and can increase a student's sense of isolation and exclusion from the community. A shift of as little as two hours, even in someone getting an adequate eight hours of sleep, can lead to increased depressive symptoms and problems with attention, concentration, and sociability.[14] Completely reversing day and night may be that much more debilitating.

Medications are less helpful in treating delayed sleep phase disorder than are treatments that target chronobiology. Bright light therapy administered upon waking in the morning is one helpful treatment strategy; another is chronotherapy.[15] In chronotherapy the student's bedtime is shifted progressively later by two to three hours each night, until a target bedtime is reached. This is an especially helpful approach for the students whose days and nights are completely reversed, but it can take as long as several weeks to work. Some more recent studies also support an afternoon or early evening dose of melatonin, combined with bright light therapy. Since melatonin is not FDA-approved, however, it's challenging to know which preparations work most reliably. In my own practice, I generally refer to a sleep clinic if a student needs chronotherapy.

Although CBT and chronotherapy are often both helpful in the same patient, sometimes one may be more appropriate than the other. Professor Leon Lack, a sleep disorder researcher in Australia, suggests that one way to decide which to emphasize is by determining whether the patient feels energetic and alert in the evening and while trying to go to sleep, or tired in the evening but alert just at bedtime, with some early morning awakening as well. If the former, then chronobiological treatment is most important, whereas CBT is more likely to help with the latter.

CHAPTER 6

Alcohol on Campus

Juan, an 18-year-old Hispanic freshman from North Carolina, avoids eye contact and squirms in his seat. His left ankle is bandaged. He's been mandated to come for an assessment following an emergency department evaluation over the weekend. He explains that he got drunk at a fraternity party, at which he'd hoped to "hook up" with a classmate. When he saw her leave with another guy, he tried to follow but fell down a half-flight of stairs and sustained an ankle sprain, as well as multiple abrasions. He admits to drinking six to seven drinks, two to three nights a week, but thinks his peers drink as much. He has had one blackout, but denies DWI charges or other consequences. "I can stop anytime I want to—but then I wouldn't have any fun at college," he says, adding that he plans to rush this particular fraternity. He's ashamed of the events of the weekend but chalks it up to frustrated love rather than alcohol, saying he's never had a girlfriend, and he can't even approach girls he likes without drinking first. Although he began drinking his senior year of high school, he never got drunk or threw up until he arrived at college. He denies tremors, cravings, or other withdrawal symptoms.

Drinking on Campus: What's "Normal"?

Most college students are legally underage for drinking alcohol, yet most do drink at least occasionally, and many drink heavily enough to make alcohol abuse a major health problem on campus. This is not a new phenomenon, but the extent of college drinking has crept up since the 1940s, and it's more concerning now that we better understand the relationship between age and alcohol use. Recent research shows that the developing brain is much more susceptible to the effects of addicting substances than the older brain. In a large, national epidemiological study of alcohol-dependent adults, 15% were diagnosable before age 18, 47% before age 21, and a full 69% of them were diagnosable before age 25.[1] Furthermore, among that majority whose addiction began before age 25, the odds for seeking help were lower than for those addicted after age 30, and the frequency, duration, and severity of alcohol dependence episodes was worse in the younger drinkers. Thus, the university setting provides a unique and critical opportunity to create positive change that can be immediate and long lasting.

Juan's drinking pattern meets the definition of binge drinking: five or more drinks in a row for men and four or more for women. The majority of accidents, injuries, and sexual mishaps related to alcohol occur among students who binge drink. Juan's impression that "everyone" drinks as much is wrong, but the numbers are in fact quite high. At four-year colleges across the country, about two in five students drink at this level, a prevalence that has remained stable over the past decade.[2]

The negative consequences of drinking appear to be on the rise. Certainly, there's greater recognition of the enormous public health burden of college drinking. Alcohol-related deaths due to unintended injury rose 3% per 100,000 between 1998 and 2005, to 1,825; this is higher than the number of student deaths due to suicide.[3] More and more students are driving while intoxicated, and in 2001, 599,000 sustained injuries related to alcohol. There's growing awareness too of just how much collateral damage is due to drinking. In 2001 nearly 700,000 students were assaulted by a drunk student, and 97,000 suffered a sexual assault or rape due to alcohol.[4] Finding an effective way to treat students like Juan is therefore critical.

Concerns about all this led the National Institute on Alcohol Abuse and Alcoholism (NIAAA) to create a Task Force on College Drinking in 1998, and since then, mounting data have prompted universities to take a more proactive stance toward dealing with alcohol misuse on campus. Research has proliferated on treatment and prevention strategies that might be most effective, and growing evidence supports early intervention. Although heavy drinking is more common in emerging adulthood than in other stages of life, the college environment itself seems to lead to heavier and more problematic drinking. Longitudinal studies show, for example, that high school students who are college bound drink less in their senior year than those not continuing their education, but both groups increase their drinking following high school graduation, and the increase is greater among college students, who surpass their out-of-school peers.[5] Students who live with their parents drink less than those living on their own, but students in campus dorms drink the most.[6] Other surveys confirm that students are particularly vulnerable to abrupt increases in alcohol use during the transition to college, even on campuses where freshmen are separated from upperclassmen.

Juan has several of the demographic risk factors for problematic drinking. Males drink heavily more than females, and Hispanic students drink more than African American students, though less than white students.[7] Juan was partying at a fraternity event and wants to rush that frat. Campuses with a strong Greek social life, or where athletic teams dominate the social scene, also have higher rates of excessive alcohol use.[8]

College students are more likely to be diagnosed with alcohol abuse than are their peers who are not in college and to drink more heavily when they do drink.[9] Although three out of every five frequent binge drinkers meet criteria for alcohol abuse, and one in five for alcohol dependence, these students lack insight: less than a quarter of them think they have a problem with alcohol.[10] Like Juan, they are unlikely to seek help on their own and often come to medical attention when someone else—a professor, family member, or dean, for example—becomes aware of the drinking through an accident or other negative consequence.

But even students who avoid binge drinking and its related immediate effects may be drinking at levels that negatively affect their long-term health. Especially problematic may be that women are unaware of gender differences in the effects of alcohol. A recent study from Mass General's Center for Addiction Medicine found that among 1,000 college freshmen attending New England schools, women exceeded NIAAA recommended daily and weekly alcohol limits about 50% more frequently than men.[11] Limits are lower for women based on physiological differences: NIAAA recommends that women drink no more than three drinks per day or seven total per week, whereas limits for men are

4 and 14, respectively. Daily drinking rates for men and women declined over the course of the first year, but *weekly* rates declined only for men. Women may feel protected by the relatively lower amounts of alcohol they consume compared to their male friends, without understanding that regularly exceeding weekly limits increases risks for breast cancer, liver disease, and other illnesses.

Assessment and Effective Treatment

Not all who binge drink in college go on to have persistent problems with alcohol later in life, but many who subsequently have lifelong problems with alcohol are represented among the heavy drinkers in college. Many colleges now implement some sort of primary prevention, such as the online curriculum AlcoholEdu. This three-hour course, when administered to all first-year students, has shown promising but short-lived results: alcohol consumption and related negative consequences are reduced, but this seems most pronounced in the 30 days following administration of the program.[12] Nevertheless, efforts at changing the culture of drinking on campus are an important step in helping students. More and more campuses are trying to do so as a way to stem the public health problems that arise from it.

Still, interventions aimed at the culture and the university community are not sufficient when an individual—like Juan—presents with significant alcohol-related difficulties. Given the pervasiveness of heavy drinking, the limited insight of the students, and the time constraints on college counseling centers, what's a psychiatrist to do when Juan comes for an appointment?

The starting point is a comprehensive assessment that determines whether he has alcohol dependence, which would require referral for more specialized treatment. A substance abuse assessment should be part of every initial intake with college students, but especially with Juan's presentation, clarifying number of drinks, frequency, and any consequences of drinking (blackouts, injuries, DWIs, headaches, etc.) becomes vital. When students are vague about the number of drinks, I guess high: "Do you drink a case of beer when you're out? No? Eight beers? Six shots?" Usually they then come up with their own estimate, which might be on the low side. The CAGE questions are helpful in this setting, as in others, for detecting dependence. Asking about alcohol use in the context of other health behaviors—smoking, exercise, nutrition, sexual practices—yields more accurate information. Asking about the student's academic functioning, relationships, emotional functioning, and triggers for drinking, or conversely, effects of drinking, is important. A thorough family history will uncover potential genetic predispositions to addiction.

The assessment also screens for comorbidities. Juan's assertion that he needs alcohol in order to approach girls might reflect a developmental issue: underdeveloped social skills, for example, or lack of experience, or perhaps feeling intimidated as a minority student living away from home for the first time. But it may also signal social anxiety disorder, or perhaps a more pervasive problem with anxiety. Social anxiety disorder can present as problematic drinking in social situations. Alcohol abuse has high rates of comorbidity with many other psychiatric diagnoses, including bipolar disorder and depression.

Juan's pattern of drinking puts him in the category of "problem drinker," according to the definition set forth by NIAAA. He is already binge drinking several times per week and has suffered significant negative consequences, including a blackout and an injury that necessitated emergency department intervention. Many colleges require students with a presentation like Juan's to complete an online educational module about problem drinking, such as *AlcoholEdu for Sanctions*, designed for students who have violated school alcohol policies. A growing number of colleges use the Brief Alcohol Screening and Intervention for College Students (BASICS) program, which involves two one-hour sessions with a trained clinician, separated by an online assessment after the first session.[13] In the absence of such a program, or in addition to it, if he is willing, he would benefit from counseling, which uses some of the same principles and techniques.

Substance abuse treatment approaches used in older adults and in other settings are less likely to be effective with emerging adults. Abstinence-based models, for example, meet with resistance and less success. The research-based treatment recommendations developed by NIAAA's task force recognize that abstinence is not a realistic goal on many college campuses. Harm-reduction strategies are more beneficial. NIAAA has developed a curriculum for health care providers working with alcohol problems in college students, *The College Drinking Prevention Curriculum for Health Care Providers*, which is available for download at its website (www.collegedrinkingprevention.gov).

The clinician's attitude toward Juan is critically important. Establishing rapport and enlisting the student's interest in addressing the problem will depend on a nonjudgmental, empathic therapist stance. This is one of the cardinal features of motivational interviewing, an approach with demonstrated efficacy in substance abuse treatment of emerging adults. Against the backdrop of a therapeutic alliance, the clinician would then help Juan see the discrepancies between his desired outcome—in this case, meeting a girl he likes—and the actual outcome of drinking—ending up in the emergency department and with possible disciplinary sanctions. In using motivational interviewing techniques, the clinician remains directive and active without getting into arguments or direct contradictions with the patient. This doesn't mean we can't disagree with the patient, especially to correct factual errors. It's a matter of finding a respectful, helpful tone—even through the frustrations of working with an intelligent student who is often engaging in foolish or even dangerous behavior—in the service of ultimately helping the student himself feel empowered to make changes in his own behavior. The goal of motivational interviewing is to decrease ambivalence and to help the person arrive at readiness for change.

Juan's belief that his peers drink heavily likely fuels his own drinking. Drinking in college is most strongly influenced by peer norms, and students across the country—in large and small, private and public institutions—consistently misperceive and exaggerate how much their peers drink.[14] They tend to think other students are more permissive in their views toward alcohol consumption than they really are, and that they consume more alcohol than they actually do. These misperceptions in turn encourage drinking and discourage those who don't drink as heavily from speaking up or modeling alternative behaviors. Correcting misperceptions of social norms has been shown to positively affect student drinking. Providing Juan with the data that show him the truth about drinking patterns at his own college will likely moderate his own drinking.

Brief interventions that combine motivational interviewing, social norms information, and decisional balance exercises work well in reducing both the frequency and the quantity of alcohol consumption in college students as well as alcohol-related problems.[15] Individual, face-to-face interventions incorporating the approaches above show the greatest improvements. This means that every interaction between a student and a clinician—even the brief medication management follow-up visit—is an opportunity to provide some intervention for excessive alcohol use.

Treating Comorbid Problems: What to Treat First?

Juan admits that he was very shy in high school, and that since arriving at college, he has felt particularly self-conscious. Frequently his heart pounds and he feels chest constriction just walking across campus, especially if he notices classmates congregating nearby. He avoids raising his hand in class, and recently when called on, he experienced tachycardia, tachypnea, dry mouth, and stammering. He has avoided returning to that class, and subsequently, having fallen behind, is considering dropping it, even though its subject interests him.

The psychiatrist discusses her clinical impressions that he is likely experiencing social anxiety disorder and recommends treatment with a serotonin-reuptake inhibitor. She continues to recommend that he reduce his drinking and explains that avoiding alcohol is especially important if he takes psychotropic medications. He says, "Doc, I can say I won't drink, but realistically, it's impossible to promise that on this campus."

Not only is alcohol abuse common among people with social anxiety disorder, but studies suggest that social anxiety significantly interferes with efforts to reduce drinking. Diagnosing social anxiety in the context of heavy drinking is somewhat more straightforward than diagnosing a comorbid mood disorder, since the fear of social interaction or social scrutiny that is a cardinal feature of social phobia is not part of alcohol addiction or withdrawal in the way that mood changes can be.

Ideally, Juan would stop drinking before starting a medication trial. However, since abstinence is not a realistic goal for him on campus, and since there's evidence that treating the social anxiety may reduce drinking and the harm related to drinking,[16] I would treat concurrently. Juan might be more open to treatment that can help him overcome his fears of talking to women than he would be to treatment targeted toward reducing drinking. Within the context of a strong therapeutic alliance, he can learn to understand the connection between the two. He might be willing to engage in an "experiment" in which he agrees to abstain from alcohol for a few weeks—or perhaps cut back by half—as he starts antidepressant medication. Extensive psychoeducation about the risks of drinking while taking a psychotropic medication is an important component of Juan's treatment, but it's likely that the potential benefits would outweigh these risks. CBT or group therapy to address the social anxiety is also an important component of the treatment. Therapy is often an excellent alternative to taking medication; however, in my experience, students with a presentation like Juan's are reluctant to participate in those forms of treatment, or find it easier to engage in them once their anxiety is at least somewhat attenuated through the use of medication.

Some students who drink heavily nonetheless voice great reluctance to the option of "putting a medicine in my body." In those instances, a nonjudgmental psychoeducational approach can go a long way toward helping the student make more rational, healthier choices. Traditional abstinence-based substance abuse treatment models have also discouraged patients in recovery from relying on other medications, but the harm-reduction model favors treatment modalities that bring about recovery and reduced risk.

Treatment decisions can become more complex when alcohol abuse is comorbid with major depressive disorder or bipolar disorder. Untreated mood disorders lead to heavier and more problematic drinking. Conversely, alcohol abuse worsens mood disorders, may actually trigger them in susceptible individuals, and is a risk factor for harm, including both suicide and violence. The DSM-5 lists substance-induced mood disorder as a rule-out diagnosis in patients presenting with mood dysregulation, so in theory it makes sense to suggest a period of abstinence, ideally a month or so. Sometimes students agree to this, but in my experience it's more common for them to simply drop out of treatment while continuing to drink, or to shop around for another provider. Students do those two things in many other circumstances as well, but the combination of alcohol abuse with many psychiatric diagnoses is so highly dangerous that as treating clinicians, we must examine our own attitudes toward integrated treatment, our training, and the current literature, and then tread lightly along a treatment path that truly does the least harm and has the highest odds of helping the student.

There are very few studies specifically in the college population to guide us. Mounting evidence supports simultaneously treating comorbid alcohol and psychiatric problems in the population at large and in adolescents. A careful history occasionally uncovers whether mood symptoms preceded alcohol use, but more often it's difficult to parse. Several studies have shown that primary mood disorders are more common than substance-induced mood disorders among those abusing alcohol, especially for women.[17] In the past, many of us were taught to treat comorbid alcohol problems and mood disorders either sequentially (treating the primary disorder first) or in parallel (treating both at the same time, but in separate settings). More recent evidence suggests that integrated treatment—treating both conditions at once, in the same setting—is most effective, both in adults and in adolescents.[18]

For students with unipolar depression and alcohol abuse, good evidence on best treatment practices is lacking. Many of the existing studies of substance abuse and mood disorder comorbidity in adults focus on alcohol dependence, rather than the alcohol abuse much more commonly seen on campus. Extrapolating from the results seen in these studies, however, and from some other studies in adolescents, both pharmacotherapy and psychotherapy appear quite beneficial. In adults, current evidence supports treating with an antidepressant, even if the person is still drinking.[19] In adolescents, fluoxetine improved both depression and substance abuse, but because the studies were small and the rate of prescribing antidepressants to teenagers has mushroomed in advance of available evidence in the past decade, the study authors declined to make treatment recommendations.[20] But the emerging adults in college are not adolescents who live at home. The selective serotonin-reuptake inhibitors, mirtazapine, venlafaxine, and other older drugs have all shown efficacy in safely reducing depressive symptoms even in alcohol-dependent patients, thus any of these are reasonable choices for emerging adults. One recent controlled trial showed that combining an SSRI (sertraline) with an opioid receptor antagonist (naltrexone) improved both depression and alcohol dependence.[21] Cognitive behavioral therapy and some other forms of psychotherapy also show benefits, especially in combination with medications.

Bipolar disorder is less commonly encountered on the college campus, but it has even greater rates of comorbidity with alcohol problems. At least one epidemiological study found that people with bipolar disorders have higher lifetime prevalence rates of alcohol abuse or dependence than people with any other psychiatric diagnosis, and other studies show that age of onset of bipolar disorder is earlier—20, on average—for alcoholics than for those with primary bipolar disorder who don't drink.[22] Alcohol abuse worsens the course of bipolar disorder and increases suicide risk. Yet most college students are unaware of the relationship between the two.[23] An essential part of the treatment is educating the student about the significant overlap and the importance of aggressive treatment of alcohol abuse in improving the outcome of bipolar disorder treatment.

Because there's such overlap in symptoms between alcohol intoxication, alcohol withdrawal, and bipolar disorder—and because the bipolar disorders present across a spectrum—making an accurate diagnosis can be challenging, especially in college students, in whom sleep deprivation and impulsivity are more common. If a student does have alcohol abuse complicating a bipolar disorder, there's evidence that the anticonvulsant mood stabilizer divalproex sodium is effective in both controlling mood symptoms and reducing alcohol-related problems.[24] Again, studies were done in alcohol-dependent adults, not in college students with somewhat different patterns of alcohol abuse, but in dependent bipolar patients, divalproex sodium reduced alcohol withdrawal symptoms and number of heavy drinking days as well as increasing time to relapse. The other anticonvulsant mood stabilizers may also be helpful—there simply isn't as much data on them; lithium appears to work less well in the comorbid population. Psychotherapy to help students cope with having a chronic illness is also invaluable in this group, as are behavioral therapies that focus on treating the alcohol use and on adherence to treatment more generally.

CHAPTER 7

Non-alcohol Substance Abuse on Campus

Do any of your counseling centers/health centers currently provide buprenorphine treatment to students? We're unfortunately seeing more and more students with opioid dependence at our college, and are starting to think about providing this at some point within the next year or so.

This query recently appeared on a list-serve of college psychiatrists to which I belong, and it generated a flurry of responses. The specialized training and legal requirements that govern treating narcotic dependence would have been considered beyond the scope of care of college counseling centers in the recent past, but clearly that is changing. Opioids are by no means the most commonly encountered drugs of abuse on campus, but this query highlights one end of the spectrum of substances that become problematic for college students. Although alcohol continues to be the most widely used substance, students also experiment with everything from illegal drugs, including marijuana, cocaine, hallucinogens, and heroin, to nonmedicinal use of legal drugs, including narcotics and stimulants. For a sizeable minority, these experiments cause significant mental health problems.

Marijuana

After alcohol, marijuana continues to be the most commonly used drug on campus. According to the 2012 National College Health Assessment, 17% of students had used marijuana in the past 30 days. The Monitoring the Future Study, which reported that annual use in college students had slightly declined in 2010 to about 33%, also cautioned that the downtrend might be about to reverse, since in 2010 marijuana use in grades 8, 10, and 12 increased. Students who are frequent users consider it less harmful than alcohol and are skeptical that it affects their academic performance or contributes to other problems. The evidence shows otherwise. Marijuana users have lower GPAs than non-users, and frequency of use correlates with GPA, with more frequent users having lower GPAs than periodic users.[1] Regardless of frequency of use, marijuana users report more psychiatric problems, including depression, anxiety, hostility, interpersonal sensitivity, and paranoia, than their peers who abstain. In a large prospective study of more than 1,000 people followed from birth to age 38, those who used cannabis four or more days a week showed a decline in IQ, impaired neuropsychological functioning, and observable attention and memory deficits as described by those who knew them best.[2] The IQ decline was greater for adolescent-onset users than for adult-onset users, and in the adolescent-onset users quitting didn't fully restore their functioning within the subsequent year. Legalization initiatives may mean that we see growing numbers of students using marijuana.

Rosa is a 23-year-old African American first-year law student, referred to the psychiatrist for a medication evaluation. She'd come in to the counseling center after panicking on exams at the end of first semester, and she'd performed poorly compared with her previous high performance in college. She reported having a hard time in law school, noting decreased focus, trouble remembering the vast amounts of material she was expected to memorize, nervousness, and significantly lowered self-esteem. She felt hopeless about improving. She wondered if she'd chosen the wrong career or perhaps too demanding a program. In the course of her intake with the counselor, she'd admitted that she was smoking a joint every night to get to sleep. She spoke of this in a quiet voice, with downcast eyes. She admitted that she'd tried quitting at the start of law school, knowing it might affect her future career, but found she felt even more restless and irritable. Smoking pot was the only time she felt relaxed, and the only way she could get to sleep at night. She'd smoked some in college, but sporadically. Her usage increased after a summer internship abroad in South Africa.

Students almost never present to counseling centers requesting treatment for marijuana dependence. It's a problem that's generally uncovered during the substance abuse assessment portion of the intake. Many have heard that cannabis is not addicting in the way other drugs are, and most believe they can stop using any time they wish. Cannabis withdrawal was not included in the DSM-IV. However, the marijuana that is currently available is more potent than that of a generation ago—sometimes 25 times as potent!—and in general, rates of dependence and other related problems have been rising in the United States and elsewhere.[3] In my clinical experience students occasionally report an increase in their use after smoking marijuana obtained abroad during semester or summer travel experiences.

DSM-5 added cannabis withdrawal as a diagnosis. There's mounting evidence not only that a withdrawal syndrome exists, but that adolescents and young adults are particularly vulnerable to it.[4] Furthermore, in the last 20 years, neurobiological research has shown that the endocannabinoid system plays an important role in the brain's developmental processes, including cell proliferation, migration, and differentiation, so that changes in its activity during stages of high plasticity, such as adolescence, may have enduring neurobehavioral sequelae.[5] Students, however, are not often open to receiving all this information.

In the vignette above, Rosa is describing symptoms of cannabis intoxication as well as symptoms of withdrawal when trying to decrease use, but she attributes all of these to the stress of law school rather than to substance dependence. The effects of cannabis withdrawal now described in DSM-5 include sleep difficulties, anxiety or restlessness, irritability, depressed mood, physical symptoms (such as abdominal pain, sweating, fever), and craving for marijuana. Interestingly, in adolescents the duration, amount, and frequency of use do not appear to correlate with withdrawal symptoms: all teens abstaining from marijuana in a small prospective study experienced withdrawal symptoms.[6] Typically these begin a day or two after abstinence and can continue for two to four weeks in adolescents and young adults, leading to a very high rate of relapse.

The attention, concentration, and memory problems plaguing Rosa are all reported consequences of cannabis use. Within 12 to 24 hours, most people experience deficits in attention, executive functioning, and short-term memory;

with chronic use, these can persist up to a month after discontinuation.[7] This means that students who have tried quitting for even a couple of weeks and noted no difference may be hasty in drawing conclusions about the drug's lack of contribution to their problems. Cannabis use is also clearly associated with an increased risk of psychosis,[8] though this is less commonly encountered among university students than are the sorts of problems Rosa describes. Students experiencing academic difficulties (especially after increased marijuana use) are usually receptive to information that helps them understand the link, and they are then more likely to be open to cutting back or eliminating marijuana use. As with alcohol, motivational interviewing and cognitive behavioral techniques that focus on harm reduction are helpful. In contrast to alcohol users, college students who use marijuana and who have experienced academic or mental health problems are more likely to want treatment.[9] The challenge is in reaching those students who believe their grades have not suffered, or students with significant comorbidities, such as depression or anxiety disorders, who feel best when they are high.

The focus on psychoeducation and on encouraging Rosa to treat her cannabis dependence cannot exclude the many other issues this vignette brings up, which are part of the complex presentations we see when working with university students. Rosa's loss of confidence in the first year of law school is not unusual, and she needs support making the adjustment to a demanding and sometimes invalidating academic environment. Her status as a female of color within a profession that has traditionally been dominated by white men may contribute to anxiety and lowered self-esteem. Since she started law school soon after an internship in South Africa, issues around oppression may have been on her mind, but she may lack opportunities to process these at school. It's important to broach these possible concerns in an empathic and supportive manner to determine if they play a role in her symptoms, in addition to focusing on the marijuana use. And of course, she may have a comorbid mood or anxiety disorder. If that is the case, concurrent treatment, as described in chapter 6, can significantly improve her outcome.

In addition to the increased potency of regular marijuana, in recent years many college campuses have also seen an influx of synthetic cannabinoids. Sold in head shops and online under various names, including Spice, Aroma, and K-2, these are often even more potent than marijuana and have similar effects. Systematic studies of the effects of these compounds are scarce, but anecdotal reports increasingly describe teens or young adults experiencing acute psychotic symptoms with synthetic cannabinoid use.[10] In a case series of 10 young adults without previous psychosis who became psychotic using synthetic cannabinoids, 30% continued to exhibit psychotic symptoms five months after use, suggesting that these drugs may trigger a chronic psychosis in susceptible individuals.[11] Five synthetic cannabinoids have now been banned in the United States; however, because of the variety of cannabinoid compounds, which can be mixed into "herbal incenses," other types and combinations will likely continue to crop up. These must remain on the radar of clinicians working with emerging adults.

Stimulants

> Susan, a 19-year-old Caucasian sophomore majoring in economics, is brought to the counseling center by her roommates, who are concerned that she's having "a breakdown." They say she's been really stressed with midterm exams, and this morning she was crying and "hyper" after staying up all night to study. They think she's been up for 48 hours, but when they suggest she go to bed, she becomes irritable and refuses. Susan sits tensely in the office, jiggling both legs and hugging herself. She denies any past psychiatric history and denies substance abuse, but eventually Susan admits that she's been taking her boyfriend's Adderall over the past two weeks. "Without it," she says "I would fail this econ class."

More college students today arrive on campus with a diagnosis of ADHD and a prescription for stimulants. For youth who've been properly diagnosed, these medicines offer a chance to fulfill academic potential that otherwise might have languished. Unfortunately, along with the increase in therapeutic use has come an increase in stimulant diversion and abuse. It's not uncommon for undergraduates, or sometimes even graduate students without a previous history of ADHD, to come for evaluation, complaining of attention or concentration difficulties and saying "I might have ADHD, because when I took my roommate's Ritalin, I studied much better."

College surveys suggest that between 7% and 15% of students use stimulants without a prescription, most commonly to study or stay awake.[12] About half of those students also use it to party: to counteract the sedating effects of alcohol, for example, or for an energy boost that allows them to stay out later. More students are snorting stimulants, and occasionally injecting them. These unapproved delivery methods increase the likelihood of harm. Snorting delivers the drug more rapidly to the brain, which raises the risk of addiction.[13] Students with ADHD are not immune to abusing their medications: they have the same patterns of recreational use described above. In addition to the risk of addiction, stimulant abuse can cause medical problems ranging from increased blood pressure to cardiac arrhythmias to sudden death. Stimulant abuse likely triggered Susan's emotional lability, or at the least contributed to insomnia, which then left her more emotionally fragile.

More psychiatrists are publicly addressing the growing problem of campus stimulant abuse. A provocative commentary in the journal *Nature* argued that the trend toward cognitive enhancement on campus by means of stimulants and other medications is not necessarily any more problematic than other human attempts at enhancement.[14] The authors expressed concerns, however, about safety and risk-benefit ratios and called for research on the effects of these drugs in healthy people, as well as policies addressing their use. An editorial in the *Canadian Medical Association Journal* in September 2011 argued that the practice of using stimulants for academic enhancement should be "denormalized" and emphasized that the vast majority of data do not support the "myth" that stimulants improve academic performance in healthy people.[15] The authors also call on universities to identify "the root cause of stimulant abuse," in essence asking the university community to recognize factors within the campus culture that encourage unhealthy attempts to boost performance.

Psychiatrists should also be aware that students who have ADHD diagnoses are often pressured to share or sell their medication. Between a third and half of students with ADHD admit to giving away or selling their stimulants;[16] it's essential to engage our patients in discussions about why this is dangerous and how to resist if asked to share. We must remain vigilant when presented with claims of lost prescriptions or requests for early refills. We must also remind our patients of the federal laws that govern distribution of controlled substances and consider employing treatment contracts that spell out these risks for students receiving stimulants. And of course, we should remain thorough and careful in accurately diagnosing and treating conditions that might benefit from treatment with stimulants. (See chapter 13.)

Other Prescription Drugs Used Recreationally
Although there's been a decline in the use of "hard" drugs, such as heroin and cocaine, on campus in the new millennium, there's been a disturbing increase in the misuse of prescription drugs. Between 7% and 9% of college students

used narcotics other than heroin in 2010, up from 2.4% in 1994; painkillers such as Oxycontin and Vicodin account for a large share of this increase.[17] These drugs also account for the increase in students seeking help for opioid addiction, as described in the extract opening this chapter. And heroin, even used intravenously, has not disappeared from campus.

There's scant information on best practices for college students suffering from opioid addiction. Most counseling centers refer out for specialized services, including detoxification and methadone or buprenorphine treatment. There's growing interest in the use of buprenorphine within the college health center setting, since this might allow students to remain enrolled in school during treatment and might encourage more students to seek and complete treatment. One study at a large northeastern university followed 27 students who presented for opioid dependence treatment at their counseling center, 63% with heroin use and the rest with prescription narcotic addiction or a combination of both.[18] Students were treated with a combination of buprenorphine, regular visits with the psychiatrist, urine drug screening, and referral for adjunctive support groups or individual outpatient therapy. Reporting a high retention rate and good efficacy and safety findings, the authors concluded that the university counseling center setting can be an appropriate and effective place to treat opioid addiction in students. As with treatment for any severe addiction, however, students should be encouraged to take a medical leave when their needs outweigh the realistic possibilities of improvement in an outpatient treatment setting.

Tobacco

Although rates of cigarette smoking have declined among college students in recent years, given tobacco's significant health hazards, there's still room for improvement. College students are less likely to smoke than their age-matched non-college-attending peers. In 2010, the 30-day prevalence rate of cigarette smoking among college students was 16%, down nearly half from a decade ago.[19] But it's very common for students to smoke when they are drinking, and many also cite it as a way to relieve stress. The rate of smoking could be higher, therefore, in clinical samples in counseling centers than in the general college population.

Most students are well aware of the health risks of smoking, so the challenge for the psychiatrist is to find a way to engage the student in a discussion of quitting without simply echoing the messages students have already heard, which they may dismiss as too authoritarian. It can be helpful to focus on triggers for smoking, and on effects of smoking, while also employing motivational interviewing techniques that allow students to define the ways in which smoking is causing problems in their lives. As with other substances, uncovering comorbid mental health issues and properly treating those may attenuate the student's interest in tobacco, but it's important not to neglect this addiction while focusing on the other targets of treatment.

Other Drugs

Students use a host of other drugs, and trends in use fluctuate. For example, MDMA, or Ecstasy, use dropped from 9.1% to 3.1% in college students between 2000 and 2009, but in 2010 the rate of use increased, not only in college students but in younger adolescents, suggesting it may be making a comeback.[20] The most common of the "club drugs," Ecstasy is used by college students who are more likely to use other illegal drugs, such as cocaine, LSD, heroin, or inhalants.[21] Web sites exist that promote its mood, sociability, and energy-enhancing effects, while downplaying its negative consequences. Sometimes these same sites also promote "herbal, legal" substances with similar effects. New psychoactive drugs seem to appear every year.

The Internet is allowing college students to access an ever-expanding variety of mind-altering substances, not all of which are illegal. These include *Salvia divinorum*, a hallucinogenic herb that can cause a brief intense high and disorientation,[22] and other substances, such as "bath salts" which are not intended for the bath by any means. The latter contains the synthetic designer drug methylenedioxypyrovalerone, which inhibits dopamine and norepinephrine reuptake and acts as a central nervous system stimulant.[23] These substances can trigger various physical symptoms, which can lead to emergency department visits, but also many psychiatric symptoms, including panic attacks, hallucinations, agitation, and self-harm. The Drug Enforcement Agency has recently banned many of these preparations, but as is the case for synthetic marijuana, manufacturers will likely tweak the formulations and continue to offer variations on them.

Remaining current on all the latest synthetic drugs available to our students is difficult. What's important is to ask students about all drugs they may be taking, even ones they consider legal and therefore safe, and to look up the ones we haven't heard of to see whether they may be contributing to psychiatric symptoms in our patients or interfering with a treatment.

CHAPTER 8

Loneliness and Relationships on Campus

Jason, a 19-year-old Caucasian sophomore from New Jersey, comes in at the urging of his parents, who are concerned about his casual talk of suicide during their weekend visit. Jason appears to find the evaluation annoying and insists there's nothing "psychiatric" wrong with him—just "unhappiness." He clarifies, "I only said I'd kill myself if things don't improve—it's nothing I'm planning to do tomorrow, or even this year. But I'm 19, Doctor, and I've never had a girlfriend. I've tried but girls never want to go out with me. I mean, people don't actually go out on this campus—they just hook up at parties, and I can't even do that right. And if I'm gonna be alone for the rest of my life, what's the point?"

Erik Erikson identified intimacy versus isolation as the core developmental task of early adulthood, and Jeffrey Arnett's theory of emerging adulthood likewise highlights the importance of relationships during this life stage. Yet for some college students, being surrounded by hundreds or thousands of their peers without forging the kinds of connections they crave only intensifies a sense of loneliness. This can lead to or exacerbate mental health difficulties. Teasing apart the psychiatric symptoms and the developmentally normal struggles can be tricky.

In college students, loneliness is associated with depression as well as with poorer physical health.[1] Although loneliness is part of the human condition, in working with students, we need to understand how it might look in this population, what the campus contributors might be, and how to help students mitigate it. The campus social landscape has been changing rapidly in the last few decades, as technology and changing social norms alter relationship templates. The increased diversity on campus both normalizes difference and creates new pockets of isolation and loneliness. Students from underrepresented racial, ethnic, religious, or socioeconomic groups, LGBT students, and the growing number of international students continue to feel outside the mainstream sometimes, despite administrative efforts on many campuses to create inclusive and diverse campus communities.

The college campus can be both a relational playground and a somewhat bizarre place. Eighteen-year-olds leave a world in which people of all ages and backgrounds interact to immerse themselves in another, where almost everyone is their age and pursuing similar goals. The potential for connection seems unlimited, but so does the constant comparison. At highly selective colleges, students who have survived intense academic competition to gain admission may find themselves facing social competition as they try to enter fraternities, sororities, or other selective living groups. Students who were admitted for their academic or extracurricular achievements may discover that their intellectual capabilities have outpaced their emotional or social skills. Campus outreach programming often focuses on sexual health—as with condom distribution programs, for example—but less on relational intimacy. As students explore and solidify their identities and interests, relationships ebb and flow.

Attachment theory provides one useful lens for understanding the types of difficulties students might experience. Not surprisingly, those who enter college with secure attachments tend to experience less loneliness than do those whose attachment patterns are either anxious or avoidant.[2] Students with insecure patterns of attachment exhibit specific social skills deficits. Even when controlling for depression, freshmen who enter college with attachment anxiety—or a tendency to cling fearfully to relationships—tend to have problems with their sense of social self-efficacy, while those who enter with attachment avoidance distance themselves from others by avoiding the self-disclosure necessary for intimacy.[3] Both these patterns lead to increased loneliness and can lead to depression. Helping a distressed student begin to see these patterns when they occur, and focusing on social skills acquisition and self-compassion, can be extremely helpful even for the students who are simply going through a developmental challenge. For the students who enter college with untreated or undiagnosed depression, social anxiety, or an eating disorder, making new friends can be particularly difficult, and a compassionate review and focus on building supportive networks is critical to their recovery.

In the vignette above, Jason's cynicism and somewhat hopeless view of the future are red flags for possible depression. But he also refers to some of the cultural elements of current campus life that make relationships even more challenging for emerging adults in college.

The "Hook-Up" Culture

Traditional dating is on the decline among emerging adults. College students have been lamenting this in my office for the past 15 years. It's confirmed by everything from the news to current TV shows, such as *Gossip Girl*, to books, including Kathleen Bogle's *Hooking Up: Sex, Dating, and Relationships on Campus*. Instead of a stepwise ritual in which potential romantic partners get to know each other emotionally and progress to physical intimacy, "hooking up" implies physical intimacy between two people who have not made any romantic commitment to one another and who may not know each other well—or at all. Students admit that "hooking up" is a purposely ambiguous term, which in part accounts for its popularity. It can imply anything from kissing to fondling to oral sex to sexual intercourse; the vagueness clouds not only the details of what actually transpired, but also the expectations of what, if anything, will follow between the two who hooked up.[4]

It's a ubiquitous phenomenon on campus, with half to three-quarters of college students reporting having hooked up in the past year.[5] It has surpassed dating as the romantic default among heterosexual college students.[6] Comparable data are harder to come by for the LGBT community. And although older generational gender stereotypes might make clinicians assume that men hook up more frequently than women, there is actually little difference in the proportions of men and women who do so.

Alcohol often plays a role in hook-ups, especially for women, and can be a predictor not only of whether a hook-up will occur, but of how "far" the encounter will go, including a greater likelihood of intercourse.[7] Caucasian students appear to hook up more than students of any other ethnicity, with the exception of those who self-classify as "multiracial."

Interestingly, one study of over two hundred students at a southern public university found that the great majority of both men and women prefer traditional dating, given the choice, especially if they are at all interested in the other person as a relationship partner, but women have a stronger preference for dating than do men.[8] A smaller minority of women (2%) compared with men (17%) have even a "slight preference" for hooking up. This study also found that men and women agree on the benefits of hooking up: they find it fun and exciting, and they like the "no strings attached" quality. But men more frequently found hooking up "sexually gratifying" than did women.

Hooking up can have various health consequences, especially when alcohol is involved. There's a greater risk of nonconsensual sex. It's more common for spontaneous sex to not include protection, putting students at risk of pregnancy or sexually transmitted diseases. Most students seem aware of this, but it doesn't necessarily affect their behavior. Studies suggest both positive and negative psychological consequences of hooking up. For example, in a small prospective study of college students, those who reported more depression and loneliness at baseline actually experienced a lessening of both after a hook-up.[9] However, the converse was also true: the students who at baseline were less lonely and depressed seemed to feel more so after hooking up.

> Jason goes on to complain that his loneliness has been especially bad since being cut from his fraternity of choice during rush week. Although he pledged another fraternity, he sees it as less socially desirable. "I think part of why I didn't get into my top choices was because I don't drink a lot, and I'm not seen as cool," he says. "And girls only wanna hook up with the jocks and the cool guys."

Media stereotypes of young adults have shifted from the traditional gender pigeonholes, which used to portray women as more interested in relationships (both friendships and romances) and men as more interested in casual sex. These days the stereotype seems to be that *everyone* is interested in casual sex. As described in the book *Hooking Up*, however, there is still a double standard in how men and women are viewed if they have frequent casual sex. It continues to be a badge of honor for men while still potentially damaging to a woman's reputation. Some young men I've worked with are tormented by depressive ruminations about whether the woman they love has had more sexual partners than they. Despite ideas of sexual equality, some old clichés seem to persist and cause real suffering as students navigate romance. Students also frequently express a desire for emotional intimacy, but are perplexed about how to seek it, since dating seems old-fashioned. They also seem to especially fear the vulnerability they must endure if they express genuine romantic interest in someone else.

As with other socially informed behaviors, such as drinking, the perception that "everyone is doing it" may in turn influence hooking-up behavior. A social norms approach, both at the individual level, when working with students, and at the campus-wide level, in outreach programs, can be enormously helpful. The Duke Social Relationships Project, which surveyed more than 4,000 Duke undergraduates over a four-year period, found that although dating was not as common as hooking up, a significant percentage of students (36% of women and 34% of men) were in fact in long-term, committed romantic relationships, and nearly 75% of all single women and men expressed a wish to be dating more.[10] Although in this study, students who drank heavily did have higher levels of "sociality," including more friends, more hook-ups, and more dates, only a minority of students actually fell into this category. So Jason falls more squarely into the mainstream at his college than he thinks he does with respect to not drinking and not dating as much as he wishes.

Giving students correct information about actual numbers, and clarifying the wide range of behavior implied by "hooking up," can mitigate some of the sense that a student like Jason has of being doomed to social exclusion. However, Jason also expresses unfortunate truths about social cachet on campus. Perceived physical attractiveness continues to be the central factor by which women are judged by men seeking a hook-up, while for women, a man's status as desirable rests on attractiveness, athletic prowess, and fraternity membership.[11] Despite the efforts of adults to encourage students to value a range of options across the many available fraternities and sororities, in my experience students continue to create social hierarchies in which some strings of Greek letters are more desirable than others. Interestingly, this can vary from campus to campus: the cool sorority on a California campus may not "make quota" on an East Coast campus, leading to much heartache for its members.

Hardest of all for students like Jason, who may lack self-assurance or advanced social skills, is that progressing to a hook-up relies largely on nonverbal cues, such as making eye contact, as well as flirting, joking, and in general being able to hang out for a long time in a relaxed manner.[12] In clinical work with students like this, any depression or social anxiety should first be addressed and treated, so that the student can then make better use of therapy that focuses on relational skills. Often group therapy is the most effective intervention, since the pattern of social difficulties may emerge in group, giving the student an opportunity to target it in the moment. The group can also normalize the often universal frustrations and fears that the student has about social interactions. As clinicians, we often have to shift our own bias from individual toward group treatment in order to effectively recommend it to our students.

In addition to individual and group therapy, less traditional treatment modalities can affect campus climates regarding hooking up and social relationships. On our campus, we've offered workshops and "retreats" on romantic relationships. Psychologist Gary Glass developed a "How to Fall in Love" series, presented outside the counseling center, which sparked interesting conversations about intimacy. Counseling center staff often join other campus groups in promoting campus-wide advocacy campaigns that encourage authenticity and expression of vulnerability, or larger conversations about hooking up and dating. Best is when students themselves are involved in the design and presentation of these programs for their own communities.

Facebook, Social Networking, and Other Digital Interactions

College students are "digital natives." They've never known a world without computers, video games, and cell phones. Much of their social life incorporates the virtual world. Even when engaging in real-world interactions, they're often also planning how to photograph and post personal updates on Facebook, or tweeting, or checking for texts about other social options. When students say they "talked" with a friend, they often mean "chatted" on a social networking site or via some other electronic mode of communication. With so much information available and constantly updated, it's easy for people to feel both more engaged and more excluded.

Because the use of social networking sites has mushroomed relatively recently—Facebook only started in 2004—there's little quantitative research on its effects on relationships and mental health. One survey of technology use in over 2,000 undergraduates at 40 randomly chosen colleges across the country found that although the majority of students felt more connected, 14% felt a greater sense of isolation due to social networking sites.[13] The same study found that although most students believe face-to-face interactions are the best way to resolve conflicts, many nonetheless have arguments entirely via text message— even though they also admit to frequent uncertainty about how to read the subtler meanings in texts. Students spend a lot of time tracking one another's sites, frequently feel compelled to immediately respond to text messages, and spend a fair amount of time analyzing the meaning of not receiving a rapid response in return. An alarming number of students—nearly 70%—have read messages online that seemed to them like a cry for help from an emotionally distressed peer.

Students increasingly express unhappiness or ask for support online. In fact, online status updates can uncover psychiatric symptoms that the poster may be reluctant to disclose elsewhere. One study of college student Facebook profiles found that 25% displayed depressive symptoms over the course of a year, and 2.5% met DSM-IV criteria for major depression based on their postings.[14] Some mental health professionals have suggested that colleges somehow monitor students' online writings for signs of distress, though the logistics of this seem impossible. It is increasingly common, however, for comments made online to make their way into the psychiatrist's office. Some students bring transcripts of online conversations, or forwarded e-mails, or saved chains of text messages. These can be helpful in understanding the student and in responding therapeutically. Occasionally a student's interpretation of social networking comments provides clues to an emerging psychosis—such as seeing unrelated posts as directly speaking to him. While this is an extreme case, it's not uncommon for students to admit to misunderstanding social cues and intentions in online interactions.

Social networking sites can also be forums for bullying and intimidation. In the highly publicized case of the freshman at Rutgers University who filmed his roommate's same-sex sexual encounter and posted it online, the student was convicted of criminal charges after the exposed roommate committed suicide. That particular case illustrates how a complex and volatile mix of social difficulties, bias, fear, and mental health issues in two college students can be stoked by the ambiguities of technology until it ignites in tragedy. Much less extreme versions of this happen every day: college students' posts are peppered with obscenities, sexual references, and sometimes racial, ethnic, and homophobic slurs. While these are interactions that have likely always happened in verbal exchanges between students, the permanence and ease of dissemination of such messages online makes their consequences potentially much more damaging to students who feel targeted and can lead to more serious judicial board disciplinary action or legal trouble for those posting. Students on both sides of these problems often present to counseling centers in distress.

In my clinical experience, when a student's online life is significantly more active than her flesh-and-blood social experience, that student's emotional balance has often tipped toward depression or another psychiatric issue. It's controversial whether the excessive use of the Internet constitutes a behavioral addiction, distinct from other mental health problems. This is a new area of research. Some studies suggest that excessive social networking use has similarities with other addictions, including a sense of losing control, neglect of personal life, mood-altering properties, tolerance, and attempts to cut back as well as to hide the behavior.[15] It's unclear how much the medium of the computer contributes to this. Regardless, it's helpful to directly address these questions when working clinically with students, especially those who report that time online is interfering with their concentration and ability to perform academically or socially. As public disclosure in online communities becomes commonplace, it may be that students become more comfortable with the idea of group therapy as well. And face-to-face group therapy has a good evidence base that supports its helpfulness in young adults struggling with relationship issues.

Loneliness as a Risk Factor for Suicide

In the vignette, Jason expressed suicidal thoughts related to his sense of loneliness. A strong social network has long been considered a protective factor in suicide assessment, but it's becoming increasingly clear that among college students, feeling isolated, and especially feeling hopeless about one's social situation, may be an independent—and modifiable—risk factor. While we know that depression and hopelessness can help predict suicidal thoughts and behavior, recent research suggests that in college students, "social hopelessness" helps distinguish between students at risk and not at risk for suicide, while general hopelessness does not.[16] Social hopelessness refers to a negative cognitive style about one's likely interpersonal relationships, including the fear of never fitting in or finding intimacy, just as Jason expressed. Students who have attempted suicide cite interpersonal difficulties among their most common problems.[17] So in working with students, it's vital to assess for social hopelessness.

Loneliness and relationship difficulties also appear to be main contributors to suicidal ideation in students in other studies.[18] Helplessness in addition to hopelessness is also a factor. More recent research suggests that components in addition to friendships and romances contribute to a student's sense of fitting in. "Belongingness," which we might assume represents the other end of the spectrum from loneliness, in fact appears to describe a distinct dimension with a big role in students' sense of well-being at college, and academic engagement is a major contributor to it.[19] Thus, in working with students who feel alone or out of place, it is important to assess not only social connections, but also the quality of their intellectual experience, their satisfaction with their classes and their chosen field of study, their extracurricular involvement, and their ties to professors and other nonstudents on campus. Working therapeutically with a student like Jason to focus on his intellectual interests and other passions, and to use these as conduits to expanding his social network, may not only bring benefits on their own but may also help him find the romantic connection he craves.

Of course, these are not the only risk factors for suicide. Any mood, anxiety, or psychotic disorder must also be assessed and treated. But in addition to that treatment, or in students presenting without a major mental health diagnosis but with relationship difficulties or loneliness, attention to these factors improves well-being and may protect against self-harm.

CHAPTER 9

Perfectionism

Twenty-three-year-old Fang-Hua, a Chinese international student in her second year of graduate studies in biochemistry, is referred by the student health center after no physical cause accounted for her presenting complaints of fatigue and oversleeping. She is frustrated that the primary care doctor suggested she may be suffering from depression, since she considers her dysphoric mood to be an entirely normal and expected reaction to her poor performance in school. Her experiments haven't yet yielded publishable results. As an undergraduate at a prestigious university in Beijing, she had nearly perfect grades and exam scores. She was also an author on a publication in a peer-reviewed journal. Since starting graduate school, she has struggled with language and lab customs but insists that "everyone does." She is very dissatisfied with her first year B+/A− average. She says her career will be over before it can even start. She dreads the shame she will bring to her family if she has to drop out of the program, but fears she may be too ill to continue: recently she's been unable to keep up her self-dictated pace of spending all her free time in the lab, and her mind wanders. The harder she works, the worse her performance seems. She berates herself when she sleeps through her alarm, then skips meals to try to make up time. She has frequent thoughts that she's become worthless. She admits to setting high standards for herself, but states, "So does my adviser, and so does my father," a scientist in China whom she claims works as much as she. "They're just good at it and I'm not." When asked about social connections, she states that school is her priority right now; she keeps in touch with old friends via e-mail and Skype, and that's sufficient for her.

Jenny, a 19-year-old Caucasian freshman from Missouri and the daughter of a Christian minister, comes in at the urging of her adviser after she left a chemistry exam in a state of panic. She tearfully describes how her mind went blank, and she's certain she'll fail the class. She clarifies that she doesn't mean literally fail, but anything below an A– is a "failure" in her mind and for her family. She is despondent that she has shown herself to be "mediocre" in college, after being valedictorian of her high school class. The clinician's suggestion that her expectations may be unrealistically high is met with a Bible quotation: "But since you are like lukewarm water, neither hot nor cold, I will spit you out of my mouth!" Jenny explains that her family and her church community interpret this to mean that God will not tolerate mediocrity, even though much of humanity is stuck within it.

Many different cultural traditions, both secular and religious, encourage striving toward perfection, though it's sometimes couched as a drive toward excellence. Universities themselves use hyperbole in their mission statements and recruitment materials. There are many benefits to setting high standards and maintaining the drive necessary to work toward achieving goals; certainly both these traits are necessary not only for admission to college, but for success in higher education and beyond. But over the past few decades, there's been a growing awareness at universities of the psychologically harmful side to perfectionism. For some students, rather than driving achievement, perfectionism not only impedes progress toward their goals, but causes great suffering along the way. Those of us working in the college counseling center setting—or with emerging adult students in other settings—must differentiate between perfectionism gone awry and symptoms of depression or obsessive thoughts that might masquerade as high standards in the student's perspective.

Perfectionism traditionally referred to an intrapersonal process in which people set excessively high or unrealistic standards for themselves and appraised their progress toward those standards in an all-or-nothing, rigid fashion that equated anything short of perfection with failure.[1] Therapeutic work with perfectionists involved helping them see that since attaining excessively high goals is unlikely, this type of cognitive style is doomed to end in unhappiness or even depression. But some university students, especially those who overcame great odds to get admitted to highly selective institutions, resist this framework. Because they believe that their perfectionistic tendencies have led to productivity and satisfaction, they're reluctant to loosen the grip of perfectionism at all.

More recently, perfectionism has been conceptualized in a more multidimensional manner, incorporating both intrapersonal and *inter*personal (social) aspects, and with recognition that it can have both adaptive and harmful effects.[2] There's some controversy, however, about which aspects of perfectionism are "healthy," although there seems to be consensus about what contributes to psychopathology. The literature distinguishes between social perfectionism and self-oriented perfectionism, which refers to the tendency to set high standards, maintain strong motivation to work, and be highly conscientious. Some researchers suggest that self-oriented perfectionists are motivated more by a desire for success than by fear of failure, and that this can lead to success in everything from athletic performance to medical school. Socially prescribed perfectionism refers to the belief that others expect one to meet extremely high standards and are very critical of one's failures.[3] It can also refer to setting excessively high standards for others in one's life.

There's growing evidence that certain characteristics of perfectionism cause more psychological harm than others. Social perfectionism, combined with high measures of self-criticism, doubts about actions, and overconcern with mistakes are consistently linked to depression, distress, and increased suicide risk.[4] Maladaptive perfectionism has also been implicated in disordered eating, hopelessness in suicidal adolescents, and insomnia.[5] Among medical students, high standards and conscientiousness seem to promote healthy progression through school, but when those same traits are paired with significant self-criticism, overconcern with mistakes, and social perfectionism, there's greater distress and depression. Working hard toward one's own goals, rather than toward goals set by others (including parents), seems to cause fewer problems.

Although some who study perfectionism argue that there is no "positive" perfectionism, and that its positive characteristics are conscientiousness rather than true perfectionism, the conceptualization of adaptive and maladaptive qualities of perfectionism fits better into a stress-diathesis framework, which takes into account the interactions of environment, biology, personality factors, and culture. For these reasons I find it a more helpful approach with the students for whom perfectionism is causing distress.

Like many—or perhaps all—international students studying in the United States, Fang-Hua, the student in the first vignette, is encountering acculturation stresses. It might seem entirely normal to a peer, professor, or clinician that now that she's working in a second language and is far from the support of family and friends, her performance might be different than her norm; however, she doesn't see it this way. Her perfectionism leads her to discount or minimize the impact of these stressors. She continues to view anything below top grades as abject failure, and projects this failure into the future. Although these may be common patterns among all students with perfectionism, there is an additional cultural element: in Asia compared with in the West, self-critical thoughts which focus on weaknesses and improving them seem to be more of a normative motivating factor.[6] When she was living at home, this may not have caused her problems. An overfocus on weaknesses, however, combined with an unrealistic appraisal of the possibilities at her current stage of training, are clearly interfering with her progress now. And in fact, self-critical perfectionism is linked with psychological and academic difficulties across cultures, both in the United States and in international populations.

Although perfectionism itself may not lead to depression under normal conditions, under high-stress conditions, including the combination of acculturation challenges and the pressures of graduate school, it may be the final ingredient that tips a student like Fang-Hua into full-blown depression. Especially difficult in Fang-Hua's presentation is that the lab she works in, and perhaps the graduate program she is part of—and even the national scientific community, in which reduced funding for research has led to greater competition for scarcer resources—all may reinforce a culture of perfectionism. Sometimes trying to therapeutically intervene with a student who is experiencing the negative aspects of perfectionism in the university setting is like doing trauma work with a person still living within a combat zone.

Taking into account all the complexities of the university context allows the clinician to build a stronger, more effective therapeutic alliance with Fang-Hua. In her experience, hard work and overachievement have in fact led to success, so she'll be wary of any approach that appears to encourage relaxed standards. She'll likely be more open to a discussion of the effects on performance of being in a foreign country. She might benefit from being encouraged to connect with other international students who share her concerns, and who can normalize the pain of leaving behind her home country. In fact, studies suggest that for Asian international students in particular, it's more helpful to focus on the effects of the stress of acculturation than on the trait of perfectionism (although both should be addressed).[7] She'd probably also be interested in data showing that treating depression or other emotional problems improves physical health and academic performance.

Of course, a full evaluation for depression and anxiety disorders, including a thorough risk assessment, is critical. It's also important to address the self-care deficits that Fang-Hua describes, which are common among students but nevertheless can be harmful. If she's expecting herself to work through meals and without sleep, she perpetuates a cycle of inability to perform, rather than the other way around. Students with high levels of perfectionism may also show greater dissatisfaction with body image or fall along the spectrum of disordered eating.

Similarly, for Jenny, the American undergraduate presented in the second vignette, perfectionism has been a part of her life, reinforced in her family and community. She has seen its rewards, so now that she's having problems, she attributes them to herself rather than to maladaptive perfectionism. The challenge in helping Jenny broaden her self-critical reactions is that she, like Fang-Hua, may view any attack on perfectionism as an attempt to compromise not only her standards but perhaps also her religious convictions. Introducing to her the concept of a continuum of perfectionism may help her recognize the ways she can diminish the debilitating effects of its maladaptive aspects while maintaining high standards.

Jenny left an exam, which suggests there may be test anxiety, panic, or another anxiety issue going on.

> Jenny admits that she is very particular about the appearance of her notes, using different colors of pen to highlight certain ideas and often recopying them at the end of the day if they don't look quite "right." In high school she used to be praised for the completeness and neatness of her notes, but in college she often runs out of time to make them look right and then finds it hard to study at all. At times when this happens she gets a sudden mental image of something terrible happening, such as seeing herself crashing into the middle lane barrier on the highway, or jumping from the bridge near campus. She insists she doesn't want to die and would never hurt herself,

and feels "crazy" when these pictures flash in her mind. She copes by repeating Bible verses to herself. This used to calm her, but recently she's found herself feeling more agitated and afraid she might pass out.

Sometimes an overconcern with having perfect test results, or doing schoolwork "just so," occurs in students with obsessive-compulsive disorder. Excessive concern with making mistakes or significant indecisiveness can indicate obsessive ruminations. In Jenny's case the repetitive prayers she describes may be a compulsion, though it's important to distinguish that from ego-syntonic praying. A careful assessment for OCD might suggest that medication with an SSRI could be helpful. Unfortunately, students who are perfectionistic and obsessive may view the recommendation for medication as another indicator of falling short of perfection, or may obsess about the option of taking medication. Patience is key in giving Jenny correct information, and in allowing her to draw her own conclusions about the ways her current problems differ from what she's previously experienced.

In the absence of the symptoms described above, however, or of other symptoms suggesting an anxiety disorder, therapy with someone like Jenny could focus on helping her connect her fear of making mistakes, overconcern about being harshly judged, and unrealistic expectations of grades with causing poor academic performance rather than success. She might benefit from consultation with a campus minister or another professional within her faith community who can help her distinguish between religious tenets and maladaptive perfectionism. Normalizing some of her concerns within the context of adjusting to college, especially at a selective institution, may also help.

Although the two students presented here are both women, perfectionism causes problems for both female and male students, although there may be some gender differences in the specifics of how it affects students. Perfectionism likely predisposes men and women to, and may even precipitate, eating disorders, a factor accounted for by the Eating Disorders Inventory (EDI), a screening tool that measures perfectionism within a subscale. But research suggests that for women, the effects of self-oriented perfectionism are moderated by the degree of socially oriented perfectionism. Although women high in either are vulnerable to eating disorders, scoring highly on *both* is much more significant for women than it is for men.[8] Other studies suggest that male students (but not women) complain of higher levels of procrastination with higher levels of socially prescribed perfectionism.[9] Female students, on the other hand, feel more guilty if they have high levels of self-oriented perfectionism than do men.[10] This finding may help explain why some women feel they must hide the effort they put into their life, whether toward academic or social or athletic success. At Duke University, the Campus Climate Study of 2003 uncovered the phenomenon of "effortless perfection" among women. This referred to the pressure young women feel to always excel without seemingly putting any work into it, while continuing to also look good, and without breaking a sweat.

For university students, group therapy is a particularly effective way to address maladaptive perfectionism. One study of an eight-week group treatment that combined cognitive behavioral and interpersonal techniques found impressive reductions in depression and anxiety, as measured by the Beck Depression Inventory and the Beck Anxiety Index, as well reduced perfectionism.[11] Perhaps the effects of examining perfectionism with peers buffers the effects of social perfectionism. This treatment helped students focus on instilling a greater sense of satisfaction in their work, setting realistic standards, and developing flexibility around standards for self and others. They also worked on exploring the students' motivation in academic, personal, and career aspirations.

The success of group treatment suggests that outreach efforts based on the group model might have a wider-ranging effect on the pervasive maladaptive aspects of perfectionism on university campuses. Again, a focus on distinguishing setting high standards from some of the more harmful aspects of perfectionism is important. Group workshops that focus on stress reduction and ways to manage perfectionism might be offered throughout the year, but especially at particularly stressful times in the academic calendar, such as before exam periods.

CHAPTER 10

Clash of Cultures

International Students

The psychology intern on the clinical team presents a case for supervision. She evaluated Ajit, a 19-year-old man from India, who came in saying, "My professor told me to come here because I'm falling behind in class, but the real problem is I am lovelorn." He describes falling in love with Jen, a Caucasian classmate in his dorm. He's not sure that Jen reciprocates his feelings, and he has been staying up nights obsessing about whether to express himself to her to find out. He feels doomed either way: crushed if she rejects him, but terrified if she doesn't because his family back in India would never approve of dating outside his race. His parents already have a partner in mind for him back home. The intern is careful to present the cultural context of the case and has asked about norms in Ajit's community of origin. She is a bit worried, however, because Ajit did report some suicidal thoughts, without intent or plan, and looked slightly unkempt, with unshaven cheeks. He spoke rapidly and intensely about his feelings for Jen and became slightly tearful at one point, making the intern reluctant to redirect him too often into diagnostic screening questions. Still, his behavior seemed within cultural norms for a young man in love and considering breaking cultural taboos. The team supported the plan of continuing the assessment and beginning therapy.

Ajit was a no-show for his follow-up appointment and didn't respond to the intern's call to check in. A week later he was referred emergently to the counseling center by student health, where he had presented requesting insomnia medicine. The referring physician was concerned about the level of difficulty sleeping and also found it unusual that the student became tearful during the evaluation there.

As previously described, international students are increasingly common at American universities. Because they face unique challenges, including language barriers, culture shock, suddenly being a minority when they'd been in the majority back home, and lack of familiarity with the American educational system, they often have higher rates of psychological problems.[1]

When international students present for psychiatric evaluation, they've frequently been referred by someone else and are reluctant to be there. Furthermore, unless there's a match between the backgrounds of patient and provider, we're likely to notice and perhaps even be a bit intimidated by the cultural differences between them and ourselves. The limited existing data do suggest that international students differ from American students in their mental health concerns and use of counseling, with both between-group and within-group differences.

International students tend to present for counseling at lower rates than American-born students and are more likely not to return after intake.[2] Some studies show utilization rates as low as 2%, and no-show rates of over 35% after the first visit. This makes the initial evaluation an even more critical and difficult opportunity for intervention. It's important to be culturally sensitive and attuned to the student's reasons for coming in while gathering as much clinically relevant information as possible. The last is important for accuracy in diagnostic assessment in order to provide the most effective treatment recommendations. These goals can seem at odds with one another, but part of the art of assessing students is finding ways to combine them.

At Ajit's first visit, he was uncomfortable about being at the counseling center, and the intern did her best to make him feel at ease by not imposing Western beliefs about therapy on him. The intern appropriately flagged concerning mental status exam findings. It was certainly possible that the student's presenting problem represented a developmentally normal relationship issue combined with adjustment difficulties, but some risk factors strongly supported further evaluation. Yet the student then dropped out of contact, and the issues of concern did not rise to the level of breaking confidentiality and, for example, asking campus police to do a safety check on him. These sorts of dilemmas are not limited to international students, but the complexities of these students' presentations often escalate into dilemmas. And psychiatrists are often asked to consult—by deans, other mental health or medical professionals, or concerned students—without the benefit of actually getting to evaluate the patient, at least initially.

International students do present in other different ways than domestic students. Looking at 218 international students at a large New York public university compared with 222 randomly selected U.S.–born students who used services at the same counseling center over a two-year period, Sharon Mitchell and her colleagues found multiple differences in the presentations of students from abroad.[3] International students were significantly more likely than their American counterparts to have been hospitalized for a psychiatric reason, and they used crisis hours more. They were more likely to express suicidal ideation and more frequently presented problems such as grief, loneliness, and academic concerns. International students were also significantly more likely to be referred by a professor or other professional. The most common diagnoses were the same, however, for both international and U.S. students, with depression and anxiety topping the list. International students were less likely to have substance abuse diagnoses. Relationship issues rose to the top of presenting concerns in at least one other study.[4]

> When Ajit presents for psychiatric evaluation, he reports sleeping only two to three hours a night for the past week, because he can't stop thinking about Jen. His concentration is diminished, and he's missed several assignment deadlines, putting him at risk of failing two classes. He's taken his roommate's Adderall several times in an attempt to get his work done but still cannot focus. Ajit says he's come to realize that the point of life is not to worry excessively about school, but to find love. He's been thinking about sex a lot, and finally asked Jen out, but she told him she just wanted to be friends. He thinks this is because he is too sexually inexperienced and that Jen could tell and was put off. There is no past psychiatric history. Family history is negative except for his mother occasionally getting "dramatic and hysterical" and, when upset, threatening to kill herself. Mental status exam is remarkable for somewhat greasy, disheveled hair, increased psychomotor activity, rapid speech, "worried" mood, and agitated, animated affect.

Thought processes are linear but somewhat illogical. There are no perceptual disturbances and no suicidal or homicidal thoughts, though he vaguely mentions he cannot imagine living without Jen. He shows impaired insight and judgment.

With Ajit's verbal permission, his roommate is invited to join the session. The roommate reports that Ajit was "very homesick" during the first semester but otherwise seemed happy. He describes a change in Ajit's behavior over the past month, even before he took the Adderall. Ajit also got drunk for the first time around then, in an effort to be more "fun" and attract Jen. But now Jen has accused Ajit of stalking her because he shows up outside her room at all hours; she has told friends she is afraid of him. Ajit laughs this off, saying he doesn't think she means this, but the roommate does not join in his laughter. The roommate asks to speak to the psychiatrist alone and reports that several students are afraid of Ajit's "weird" behavior and have been staying away from him.

Ajit does not believe he needs counseling and is opposed to taking medications of any kind. He does not want to give permission for his parents to be contacted.

Homesickness is a normal complaint of first-year students regardless of their origin, but it is more common and more intense in international students, especially younger students who are farther away from home.[5] It has been linked to depression and anxiety. Because the differential diagnosis for Ajit must include bipolar disorder, it would be helpful to know if what his roommate considered homesickness might actually have been depression. More detailed questions can sometimes uncover that distinction, but not always.

There is also the issue of one student romantically pursuing another, uninterested student. Although Ajit is physically small and has no history of violence, Jen's fear of being stalked must be taken seriously. At the same time, it's important to be sensitive to the possibility of bias or fears born out of a lack of cultural understanding. Since the massacre at Virginia Tech especially, students and faculty seem particularly susceptible to being shaken by unusual behavior by students from certain ethnic backgrounds. Regardless, students who are worried that they're being stalked must be supported, by referral to campus resources, including police, faculty, and services to prevent sexual assault.

Sometimes both students in a pair with an allegation of stalking might present separately for treatment to the counseling center and to the same psychiatrist, in which case it's very important to be on the lookout for conflict of interest. The ideal would be to refer one of the students to another psychiatrist, if available, without violating either student's confidentiality.

Often the cultural divide between students raised in different countries leads to social misunderstandings and missteps, as courtship practices can vary widely. American culture is highly mobile and values individualism, so friendships and romances are viewed as less permanent or serious than they are in many other countries; international students may misinterpret casual superficial pleasantries as signs of sincere interest. Ajit's behavior, however, is out of step with what would be considered appropriate in his country of origin as well as in his current peer group. His impaired insight and judgment suggest that he may in fact be suffering from a mood or other psychiatric disorder rather than a developmental or adjustment problem. Collateral information from roommates, peers, professors, and family, if available, can be critical to accurate diagnosis.

Ajit had recently used more alcohol than normal for him as well as stimulants. Did mood dysregulation lead to the uncharacteristic substance use, or vice versa? A full assessment to rule out bipolar disorder, other mood disorders, and anxiety disorders is essential. But making a diagnosis brings up unique challenges in working with international students, for whom mental illness is often more stigmatized and shameful than for domestic students. The student may not have the capacity to understand a diagnosis such as bipolar disorder, or may refuse treatment. The idea that emotional difficulties can be caused by medical illnesses, which can be ameliorated through medication, may be completely foreign to the student. International students often don't want to involve their families, which poses challenges for school personnel on how to best support the student. If treatment requires hospitalization or otherwise taking time off from school, the student's visa status may be at risk, and often the student doesn't want to return home without having completed the semester or year. In these complicated situations, consultation with peers in the counseling center can be invaluable. With permission, consultation with deans, advisers, and family is also essential. Often the student has already come to the attention of deans or other administrative faculty, and these people can contact the family when there's alarming behavior or severe academic underperformance, even if the psychiatrist does not have permission to do so. A focus on the behavior of concern, without overemphasizing diagnoses, can sometimes help get through an impasse. Collaboration in the service of helping the student is key.

Of course, grouping students under the heading "international" blurs the vast cultural differences between the countries and continents from which they come. Even within a country, students coming from one family may present differently than those from another. Socioeconomic class and educational background create differences. Some international students are the children of people who themselves studied or lived in the United States at some point, and these students are thus much more acculturated than their background label might suggest. Mitchell's study comparing international and U.S. student utilization of counseling services also recognized the limitations of data on internationals; students from Hong Kong, for example, may have very different attitudes toward mental health concerns than students from mainland China, or those from Korea. Nevertheless, a good starting point is simply to be aware that differences exist between international and American students and to maintain a humble and curious attitude. We can start with trying to be familiar with as many of the general differences as possible, while continuing to learn about the finer distinctions.

It's not unusual for international students like Ajit to refuse psychiatric medications. Studies confirm that Asian students are more concerned than European or North American students about medication management. In my own clinical experience, students not only from Asia but from many countries outside the United States are more reluctant to take psychotropic medications than their American peers. Engaging them in detailed discussions about their fears, expectations, and objections is critical to helping them fully understand their treatment options, and to ultimately get them to adhere to effective treatment. College students value objective data and can often understand complex biological and pharmacological explanations of their difficulties. Unless we have concerns about safety or the student's illness rapidly worsening, however, remaining flexible in treating students from other countries can be the most therapeutic intervention. For example, one Asian student who had generalized anxiety disorder refused serotonin-reuptake inhibitors repeatedly but accepted limited low-dose benzodiazepine treatment for significant performance anxiety that was making it difficult for him to find a job. He tended to come in for "check-in" appointments, where he would describe his symptoms in great detail but then politely decline all offered therapeutic interventions. Over the course of 18 months of these infrequent but regular visits, however, he showed some improvement and became open to the idea of trying an antidepressant medication. He eventually came to trust our relationship and was willing to try a Western approach to his problems, but only after other efforts—including meditation, yoga, and talk therapy—showed only limited benefit.

Students from other countries may also be taking medications mailed to them by relatives back home, including traditional herbal remedies, pharmaceutical agents not available in the United States, or supplements. Some students drink teas with specially mixed ingredients prepared by traditional healers. These can have psychoactive properties that interact with medications we prescribe, so it's important to ask in an open-ended way about what approaches they have already tried for their problem. Simply asking whether they are taking any medication might not uncover these other substances.

Not being familiar with the conventions of psychotherapy, international students may also be less likely to adhere to weekly or bimonthly hour-long sessions, instead favoring a more episodic, come-in-as-needed approach. Although this also goes against the principles of Western psychotherapy models, it might be effective for them. We need systematic research to resolve the question, but in the meantime, it seems most important to engage them in treatment of some kind that can show evidence of improvement. At Duke we've experimented with expanding our offering of complementary treatments, such as yoga and mindfulness meditation groups, and found that these tend to be much better attended by international students. Groups that meet outside the counseling center specifically for students from various other countries can bolster support. This approach has worked at Duke and other counseling centers.[6] Outreach efforts that involve international faculty and that help students begin to understand the link between emotional health and academic performance can also be quite effective.

In this chapter's vignette, Ajit's lack of trepidation about his grades is somewhat unusual for most international students and may indicate his level of impairment. Among students seen in counseling centers, international students' concerns centered more on academic issues than did those of their American peers, even though their academic performance itself was about the same.[7] Linking treatment to academic success is therefore often a way to help make intervention more relevant and acceptable to these students, compared with focusing on personal problems or emotions alone. Other studies have found that Asian students more frequently express depressive symptoms through somatic complaints.[8] Students may thus present to student health or a primary care doctor rather than to the counseling center or a psychiatrist. When they're referred on to counseling, they may be reluctant to follow through or may feel as if their symptoms have been dismissed unless we adequately explain the rationale in ways that make sense to them.

Several studies suggest that international students prefer more directive counseling styles, peppered with advice and practical information. Students from African countries, for example, who are accustomed to more hierarchical social structures, may even view clinicians who are nondirective as incompetent.[9] American students from minority groups likewise may prefer more directive treatment approaches. As physicians who have historically been trained in a hierarchical model, psychiatrists may be more comfortable with directive treatment approaches than their non-M.D. colleagues. However, psychiatrists with significant experience working with college students know that collaborative, egalitarian models of care work better for American students. It's a delicate balance: like their American counterparts, intelligent young adults from all over the world respond poorly to overly rushed, authoritarian communication styles. Providing clear recommendations, explaining the rationale for recommended treatment, discussing alternatives, eliciting questions and concerns, all while maintaining a respectful stance toward the student has in my experience worked best with students from all backgrounds.

CHAPTER 11

Clash of Cultures

LGBT Students

In the last two decades, universities have attended to the increasing diversity among their students, which has led to greater acceptance of and attention to the needs of students from minority sexual orientations: lesbian, gay, and bisexual students. Transgender students, whose concerns center more on gender identity than on sexual orientation, are usually included within the LGBT categorization, even though their needs or issues may differ. The generation currently in college has grown up with greater visibility and acceptance of LGBT people, with openly gay celebrities like Ellen DeGeneres and Clay Aiken, same-sex marriage legal in some states, recent acceptance in the military of openly gay troops, and films and TV shows that normalize the lives of LGBT people. More and more universities feature classes and even majors that focus on LGBT studies, "queer studies," or related disciplines.

Yet research suggests that LGBT students continue to face greater discrimination and harassment on campus than do other minority groups, and that even open prejudice against LGBT students continues to be socially acceptable in a way that other prejudices no longer are.[1] Continued clashes in our society over LGBT rights, and the great variability in how acceptable these issues are within various smaller communities, affect the emotional well-being of emerging adults. Highly publicized tragedies, such as the death of Tyler Clementi because of bullying based on his sexual orientation, have drawn attention to these problems. But even in the absence of such extreme situations, LGBT students may adjust somewhat differently to college and present with mental health concerns that diverge from those of their heterosexual peers.[2] For those of us working with emerging adults, providing compassionate, affirming care can have a tremendous effect on these students.

Sexual Orientation

Bruce is a 19-year-old white freshman from Alabama who comes to the counseling center complaining of depression. He endorses low mood, anhedonia, frequent crying, and a tendency to isolate himself from his peers, but he denies any neurovegetative symptoms. His concentration suffers only "sometimes," and at first he's vague about when. He's been excelling academically. On the intake paperwork, he omits the demographic portion regarding sexual orientation and is vague in answering questions about relationships and social supports. He then asks whether any medicines can reduce sexual desire. The psychiatrist gently probes for details of the desire he wishes to avoid and of his sexual experiences. Bruce quietly admits that he's been attracted to men for years now, but as the son of an evangelical Christian minister, he fears it would destroy his family if he came out. He hastens to explain that he is also committed to the religious community in which he grew up, and is loath to lose their good opinion as well. He did attend a program at the university's LGBT center during orientation and felt further confused because he didn't identify with some of the more activist stances that other students took. It's only when he starts to think about how he might resolve this conflict in his life that he starts to obsess, and his concentration lapses. Lately he's felt hopeless about ever being happy since he "can't" be gay. At those times he's experienced helplessness, guilt, and suicidal thoughts. His fear of eternal damnation scares him away from both suicide and exploring his sexuality.

Given the highly emotionally charged clashes in our culture over gay rights, and the seemingly irreconcilable divide between some religious groups and the notion of whether sexual orientation and gender identity are "choices" or biologically predetermined, working with a student like Bruce can bring up confusion, fear, and counter-transference. What happens when a student's multiple identities clash? In attempting to remain culturally aware and sensitive, we might want to respect Bruce's commitment to his religion as well as his physi-ological and psychological need to be true to his sexual orientation. As licensed professionals (physicians, psychologists, clinical social workers, nurses), we must turn to our evidence-based knowledge and the ethical codes of our discipline—along with the principle of "first, do no harm"—to help students caught in such seemingly impossible inner conflicts.

Bruce is clearly suffering. He doesn't meet all the criteria for a major de-pressive episode, but he could have another depressive disorder or dysthymia. His symptoms appear directly related to a major developmental conflict that touches on identity, sexuality, and the capacity for intimacy. Although our diagnostic frameworks for depression are shifting away from a focus on life events in favor of symptom checklists, ignoring the sexual orientation issues in Bruce's presentation and solely targeting the depression is unlikely to be genu-inely helpful to him. This doesn't mean that we wouldn't offer him treatments for depression that we might offer another student without these additional concerns, but that we must address these other important factors in planning out his care.

Sexual minority status is a risk factor for suicide. One study found that nearly one in five gay college students has attempted to kill himself.[3] Although most emerging adults will face a crisis related to normal developmental issues dur-ing their college years, for many LGBT students, issues around sexual identity and orientation take precedence, often to the exclusion of other developmental tasks.[4] In my clinical experience, students can experience severe depressive and anxiety symptoms in the midst of a difficult coming out process, and then exhibit substantial improvement or resolution of these symptoms once they are secure within their sexual orientation and have found an affirming community. Bruce has lived with significant homophobia within his family and his community, and he has internalized those beliefs. It's critical that the clinician he sees doesn't reinforce homophobia. Too rapidly offering medication—especially antidepres-sants that might in fact lower Bruce's sexual drive—might be seen as agreeing with his stated desire to curb his same-sex attractions, unless done within the context of a sensitive, affirming exploration of sexual orientation issues.

College students sometimes come to counseling asking whether they "might be gay." Psychologist Kenneth Cohen, who specializes in working with LGBT issues at Cornell, suggests that often there's the hidden hope within that ques-tion that a therapist will "assure" the student that he's not gay; Cohen recommends first probing whether the student "really wants to know," and then asking what it might mean if he or she *were* gay.[5] Therapy can help students understand the distinct but related domains of sexuality: sexual orientation (the direction of the student's erotic thoughts, feelings, and fantasies), sexual behavior (the sexual actions that a person takes), and sexual identity (how that student, and society, "label the student's sexual feelings, attractions and behavior"). Cohen suggests asking these four questions to help clarify a student's sexual orientation:

1. To whom are you emotionally (not sexually) attracted? (Both males and females are more often emotionally attracted to females, which can confuse some women.)
2. To whom are you erotically, or sexually, attracted?
3. When alone and masturbating, which sex do you think about? (Or, which kind of pornography attracts you?)
4. When home alone and masturbating, and on the verge of coming or just after, which sex are you thinking about or looking at?

Cohen cautions that these questions are more salient for male than for female students, however, because female sexuality is more contextual and emotion based.

The process of coming out often begins with questioning and some identity confusion, during which the person's self-esteem is vulnerable because of fear of rejection.[6] The next stage is of identity comparison, followed by a third stage of identity tolerance, in which the student might begin to make contact with other LGBT students to find affirmation. In the vignette above, Bruce is still early in the first or second stage. There are three subsequent stages: identity acceptance, identity pride (during which a student might dichotomize homosexual / heterosexual identities as good / not good), and finally identity synthesis. We may see students at any stage along this spectrum. For students further along, their LGB identity is often not a focus of their presenting concern or of their counseling. Even then, sensitivity to this part of their identity enhances the therapeutic alliance.

LGBT students may experience conflict between various aspects of their identities not only around religion, but also around race, ethnicity, or country of origin. Bruce is stuck because he believes that the only way out of his dilemma is to deny one aspect of his identity. Some religious teachings do counsel that living a celibate life—or not engaging in behavior congruent with one's same-sex sexual orientation—is the only "nonsinful" approach.

> At the second session, Bruce reports that in his senior year of high school, he did confide in a youth minister at his church that he was having homoerotic thoughts and was told that it was normal in adolescent boys, and he'd outgrow it. Most important was to not act on those feelings. If the feelings persisted, the youth minister added, reparative therapy would help. Bruce says that if medicine can't curb his sexual longings, perhaps it's time for reparative therapy and asks whether the psychiatrist can refer him to a good reparative therapist. As his psychiatrist presents this case in a multidisci-plinary treatment team meeting, one of the psychiatry residents suggests that this seems a reasonable option: otherwise, the treating clinician is privileging one of the patient's identities over the others and not respecting the patient's own stated wish.

Although certain religious groups cite testimonials about people who have changed their sexual orientation through "reparative therapy," or "conversion therapy," there is no empirical evidence that it achieves its intended goals, and there *is* evidence that it can be harmful. Much of the support for its efficacy was based on a 2003 study by psychiatrist Robert Spitzer, who was considered a credible researcher. In 2012 Spitzer himself retracted his study, noting it was flawed and that he no longer believed the design actually answered its basic question.[7] Spitzer issued an apology to the LGBT community and especially "to any gay person who wasted time and energy" on this. But long before this, the American Psychiatric Association, as well as other major professional or-ganizations, including the American Psychological Association, the American Medical Association, the American Academy of Pediatrics, and the National Association of Social Workers, all issued position statements opposing any therapy that purports to change sexual orientation. In 2012 the California As-sembly passed a bill barring the use of conversion therapies in minors, again citing both lack of efficacy evidence and risk of harm to those who undergo these interventions.[8]

The psychiatry resident in the vignette needs to be educated about both the evidence and the stance that her own and other professional organizations have taken. It would be unethical—as well as unhelpful and likely harmful—to refer Bruce for reparative therapy. Bruce needs education about why his re-quest is unlikely to resolve his conflict, and assurance that there *are* effective forms of therapy, which help people try to integrate their sexual orientation and their religious beliefs, but not through changing sexual orientation. Therapy with Bruce should provide a safe space in which he can discuss his feelings and beliefs about his religious and sexual identities, fears of loss around one or both, and exploration of possible ways to integrate rather than privilege either part of his identity.[9]

In working with LGBT students, we facilitate the therapeutic alliance when we pay attention to the language we use. Because psychiatry historically classified homosexuality as a mental disorder, certain terms remain offensive to some gay people, including use of the word "homosexual." Some students find even the words "gay, lesbian, bi, or transgender" to be white social constructs of identity that may not be relevant to their own experiences; they may prefer terms such as same-gender loving, gender queer, pansexual, or others.[10] In general, following students' lead and using the same language they use is best.

Gender Minority Students

As sexual orientation issues have gained more visibility on college campuses, knowledge of and comfort with gender minority issues lag, even among faculty and counseling center staff. Students themselves are often more comfortable than the older generations on campus with a growing range of gender-atypical expression and are developing more gender-neutral forms of referring to themselves and one another. The number of college students who are out as transgender has increased. There has been a push among activists and professional organizations to depathologize people who, in sense of self or in behavior, fall outside typical male-female constructs, and to be more accepting of gender variance. The World Professional Association for Transgender Health (WPATH) published a statement in 2010 asserting, "The expression of gender characteristics, including identities, that are not stereotypically associated with one's assigned sex at birth is a common and culturally-diverse human phenomenon [that] should not be judged as inherently pathological or negative."[11] Unfortunately, violence and discrimination against transgender people persists, and some studies suggest that it may be on the rise.[12]

"Gender" and "sex," though often used interchangeably, are not synonymous. "Gender" is a broader designation than "sex," which refers to the biological indices—anatomy, chromosomes, hormones—that usually identify a person as male or female. "Gender" refers to the cultural and societal factors that make someone masculine or feminine, and usually includes sex. Most people's gender identity is aligned with their biological sex. But for others, around the world and across time, there is a mismatch. "Gender nonconformity" refers to how much a person's gender identity, behavior, or role differs from expected cultural norms;[13] it does not imply distress, although some gender-nonconforming people do experience distress. Gender identity and sexual orientation are distinct but related.

The umbrella term "transgender" encompasses various behaviors and values that transcend traditional gender norms. It can refer to people who don't identify with their biological sex and actively try to change it via hormonal or surgical treatments. It also includes people who are comfortable with their aligned gender and biological sex, but who cross-dress, or engage in activism to challenge societal gender norms and dress, behaving in gender-atypical ways. "Transgender" encompasses people who have been called transsexual, cross-dressers (transvestites), and "gender-benders." The terms "transvestite" and "gender-bender" are considered derogatory and should be avoided.[14]

Students employ a range of new terms, from gender-nonconforming, to cisgender (comfortable with the gender assigned at birth), to bigender (not wanting to identify as either man or woman), to gender queer. Some students prefer to entirely avoid gender pronouns, which can be difficult given our language's reliance on them. These students might use variations of "he" or "she," such as "ze" and "zir" as the gender-neutral equivalent of "his" or "her."[15]

There's little empirical research regarding the experiences of transgender college students, though their concerns are starting to get more attention within university communities. There *is* evidence that transgender students are subjected to more discrimination on campus than their peers who identify as either male or female, and that transgender students in both clinical and nonclinical samples experience significantly more psychological distress than cisgender students.[16]

Psychiatry's understanding of what constitutes a "disorder" regarding gender identity is evolving. DSM-IV included gender identity disorder (GID) to refer to people who did not identify with their biological gender and had a strong urge to live as the opposite gender. But recognizing the range of comfort—or difficulty—among gender-nonconforming people, and the stigmatizing nature of the GID diagnosis, the workgroup for DSM-5 proposed dropping the GID diagnosis and instead emphasizing the unhappiness that can occur when there is incongruence between one's perceived gender and one's body—usually as a result of cultural bias and oppression rather than clearly due to a psychiatric issue—via a gender dysphoria diagnosis. This emphasizes treating dysphoria, not identity, as the clinical problem. DSM-5 also separates gender dysphoria from the sexual dysfunctions and paraphilias and includes specifiers that relate to whether the person is in transition or post-transition to their desired gender, as well as whether there is a disorder of sex development, such as congenital adrenal hyperplasia.

> Alan, a 21-year-old Caucasian junior, identifies as transgender on intake paperwork and presents requesting medication for sleep. Alan begins the session tearfully noting frustration that the receptionist had used the chart name "Alice," which Alan is in the process of legally changing. The therapist asks for guidance regarding gender pronouns and notes that she will do her best to use correct names and pronouns; Alan prefers to be referred to as "he." He visibly calms down after this exchange and reports that he is in the midst of transitioning from female to male. He reports much stress around all the battles he is fighting to do this: with parents, who are unaccepting; with the university, whose records are cumbersome to change; and most recently, with his girlfriend of a year, who is threatening to end the relationship. Initially reticent when asked about medications, Alan admits that a week ago he began T, or testosterone. He is getting this through the Internet but assures the therapist that he's read quite a bit about it, has had a physical exam and bloodwork done at a mall clinic, and has friends who have transitioned and are guiding Alan's process. He is defensive and tearful, noting that he doesn't need another person telling him how to live his life, and he is guarded when asked about past psychiatric history, stating, "I've been depressed before, but now I know it's because I've been trying to live in the wrong body. I'm here just for help sleeping and then I wouldn't be so on edge." He denies manic symptoms currently or in the past. There is no history of alcohol or substance abuse. Alan did receive medical attention two years ago for a suicide attempt by overdose, but he denies current suicidal thoughts.

Many psychological, legal, cultural, and ethical issues arise in working with transgender students. A full discussion of all of these is beyond the scope of this chapter, but the vignette above illustrates a few that are not uncommon. Table 11.1 lists resources that contain more in-depth information on some of these issues.

Transgender emerging adults are at increased risk for suicide. In one study of 55 15- to 21-year-old transgender people in New York, nearly half of whom

Table 11.1   Resources for working with transgender students

Medically / professionally focused books

Principles of Transgender Medicine and Surgery, edited by Randi Ettner, Stan Monstrey, and Evan Eyler. (2007; Haworth Press).
Guidelines for Transgender Care, by Walter Bockting and Joshua Goldberg (2007; Haworth Press).

Books for mental health professionals, students, and others close to them

True Selves: Understanding Transsexualism; For Families, Friends, Coworkers, and Helping Professionals, by Mildred Brown and Chloe Ann Rounsley (1996; Jossey-Bass).
Transgender Emergence, by Ari Lev (2004; Haworth Press).
Transitions of the Heart: Stories of Love, Struggle, and Acceptance by Mothers of Transgender Children, edited by Rachel Pepper (2012; Cleis Press).
She's Not There, by Jennifer Finney Boylan (2004; Broadway).
The Testosterone Files, by Max Wolf Valerio (2006: Seal Press).
Gender Outlaw: The Next Generation, by Kate Bornstein and S. Bear Bergman (2010; Seal Press).

Web sites

World Professional Association for Transgender Health (WPATH), www.wpath.org
Gender Identity Research and Education Society (GIRES), www.gires.org.uk
How Colleges and Universities Can Improve Their Environments for TG/TS Students, by Lynn Conway, http://ai.eecs.umich.edu/people/conway/TS/College.html

Films / documentaries

Transgeneration (Sundance documentary following four trans college students); available on iTunes
Boy I Am (DVD)

were in college, 45% "seriously thought of taking their lives," another 20% "sometimes or often" had such thoughts, and 25% of them had attempted suicide.[17] Of those who had attempted suicide, all said that at least one of their attempts was directly related to being transgender. Compared with transgender youth who never attempted suicide, those who did attempt had experienced more verbal and physical abuse from their parents and had lower body esteem, especially with regard to weight satisfaction and how others view their bodies. In another study of transgender college students, three times as many who identified as transgender rather than cisgender —about a quarter, again, of the sample—attempted suicide.[18] This second study, which compared transgender students in both a clinical and a nonclinical sample, alarmingly found that even the students in the nonclinical sample reported significant distress (measured with CCAPS) and suicidal thoughts. Another study found transgender college students are wary of counseling services for many reasons, ranging from a sense that counselors are uninformed to fear of being considered "crazy" to fear of being given a GID diagnosis.[19]

Students are not comforted by counselors who profess ignorance on issues of gender identity, and yet, that's the most honest approach to take when we truly don't know. It's important to develop a list of expert referrals—psychiatrists, therapists, and medical doctors—who are knowledgeable about trans issues, and to refer as appropriate. We also need to educate ourselves about gender minority issues, through our own reading, bringing expert speakers to campus, and attending professional meetings where these topics are covered. We must constantly bring an attitude of humility and curiosity to learning about gender identity issues, especially as cultural norms continue to shift, science uncovers new information, and more students seek help with these concerns.

In working with transgender students, especially those who, like Alan, want to start or are in the process of using cross-gender hormones, it's critical to be familiar with the WPATH Standards of Care for the Health of Transsexual, Transgender, and Gender Nonconforming People (formerly referred to as the Benjamin guidelines). These evidence-based standards, revised in 2011, no longer require psychotherapy prior to the start of hormonal therapy, although a mental health screen is still required, and therapy is still recommended.[20] Alan insists insomnia is his only concern, but we must nevertheless screen for other psychiatric problems just as we would with any other patient, helping Alan understand that it's intended not to place barriers in his way but to bring relief for any co-existing problem. It's important to normalize the feelings of frustration and sadness triggered by multiple rejections (parents and romantic partner, in this case) while also helping Alan acknowledge that transitioning is a process that takes time. Counseling—or at the very least, education—can help Alan have more realistic expectations of hormonal treatment, the legal processes around name change, and future options.

If a careful risk assessment determines that Alan is at low risk for self-harm, we'd certainly focus initially on treating his insomnia, prescribing a CBT-based insomnia treatment or a short-term course of sedative-hypnotic medication like zolpidem. Some physicians might be understandably reluctant to prescribe a sleeping pill to a distressed student with a history of overdose, who likely could also benefit from treatment for depression or anxiety. However, desperation around insomnia and frustration with a perceived lack of empathy in medical professionals can present equal or even greater risk for a student like

Alan. Giving a very limited quantity of a sedative-hypnotic—even as few as five to ten tablets, without refills—while working on developing a therapeutic relationship that might allow for deeper exploration of the many stressors and issues he is currently facing might in the long run really help this student attain emotional stability.

Students sometimes circumvent established medical care in favor of Internet prescribers because either they are so frustrated by perceived obstacles to transitioning or they can't afford medical care. Current WPATH guidelines state, "It is important for mental health professionals to recognize that decisions about hormones are first and foremost the client's decisions," but that mental health professionals "have a responsibility to encourage, guide, and assist clients with making fully informed decisions and becoming adequately prepared." Has Alan been making fully informed decisions, if he is receiving hormones via the Internet? Is he adequately prepared for the potential effects and side effects of testosterone? Part of the standard of care for people receiving hormone treatment is informed consent, a step that Alan has bypassed by getting medicine online. Within the context of a caring, supportive relationship, the psychiatrist can educate Alan about the purpose of informed consent, the WPATH criteria for hormone therapy (see table 11.2), and the important information that can protect his health as he continues to transition. Also critical is a good referral to a medical doctor who is skilled in working with transgender patients.

In addition to therapy, support groups—online and off—can be helpful for transgender students. Sometimes these are available through a university's LGBT center. Transgender students who do want therapy, or who are considering surgical interventions, which require therapy first, often fall outside the brief therapy model and require referral for longer-term work (see table 11.3). In areas where culturally competent clinicians may be scarce, however, an informed counseling center clinician, or online resources, may be the best and most ethical treatment option.

Table 11.2   WPATH criteria for hormone therapy

1. Persistent, well-documented gender dysphoria
2. Capacity to make a fully informed decision and to consent for treatment
3. Age of majority in a given country (if younger, follow the WPATH Standards of Care for assessment and treatment of children and adolescents with gender dysphoria)
4. Significant medical or mental health concerns, if present, must be reasonably well controlled

Table 11.3   Goals of psychotherapy for emerging adults with gender concerns

1. Main goal: help gender-nonconforming or transgender people achieve long-term comfort in expressing their gender identity, with realistic chances for success in school, work, and relationships.
2. Explore and clarify gender identity and role.
3. Discuss impact of stigma and discrimination on student's mental health and on human development in general.
4. Facilitate coming out process, including, if applicable, changes in gender role expression via feminizing or masculinizing medical interventions.
5. Provide support, especially through helping student develop interpersonal skills and resilience.
6. Treat any identified coexisting mental health issues, such as depression, anxiety, or substance abuse.

Source: Adapted from WPATH. (2011). "Standards of Care for the Health of Transsexual, Transgender, and Gender Nonconforming People." *International Journal of Transgenderism, 13,* 165–232.

As with sexual orientation issues, a student's nationality, ethnicity, or religious background colors their feelings about their gender identity. It's important to take cultural context into account and use the best currently available clinical evidence we have in helping students achieve *general* psychological well-being, including with regard to gender identity. WPATH standards say, "Treatment aimed at trying to change a person's gender identity and lived gender expression to become more congruent with sex assigned at birth" is ineffective and unethical.

CHAPTER 12

Disordered Eating

Nineteen-year-old Nicole, a Caucasian sophomore from North Carolina, is referred by her professor for panic during an exam and general poor academic performance. She tearfully admits that she has had increasing trouble concentrating and wonders if she might have ADHD. She also reports low energy, dizzy spells, and loss of interest over the past two months. Routine screening questions on an intake questionnaire (the CCAPS) uncover a preoccupation with body weight, feelings of dissatisfaction with body shape, and a wish for thinness, but when asked about these issues in the interview, she becomes frustrated and insists, "I'm not anorexic or anything—you can see that by looking at me." She denies over-restricting, purging, or laxative or diuretic abuse. "I worry about my weight like all college women do," she states.

In fact, college women probably do worry more about weight and body image than age-matched peers who are not students and women in other age groups. As emerging adults navigate the normal developmental challenges of being in college, including consolidating identity and forming intimate relationships, they are often aware of their bodies in new ways. And their bodies often change in college. The idea of the "freshman fifteen" has become part of our cultural lexicon and refers to the weight gain students commonly experience as they navigate changes in their diet in the dorms, along with changes in their levels of activity. The cultural focus on thinness as desirable, the exposure to peers who may be overly preoccupied with food or weight, and the competitive nature of living on a college campus all may contribute to "intense" dieting or other weight-loss-related behaviors that put students at risk of an eating disorder, behaviors that one recent report found in two-thirds of college women.[1]

A continuum of disordered eating is common on campus, with the majority of problems falling into what's been called the "subclinical" range—not meeting all DSM-IV criteria for an eating disorder. That may change somewhat as the categories are broadened in the DSM-5, in recognition of the fact that the older criteria excluded some fairly ill individuals. Full-blown anorexia and bulimia nervosa, which cause serious health problems and can become life-threatening illnesses, are also more common on campus—not surprisingly, since they usually start in the adolescent years and may first be recognized in college. Although these have been considered predominantly disorders of Western white women, with prevalence rates of about 0.5% for anorexia nervosa and 1% to 3% for bulimia in the general U.S. population[2] (with men making up less than 10% of the total), that is changing. One study found that over 40% of university women in a sample in Taiwan were at risk of an eating disorder; others reported a similar spreading of disordered eating concerns among university women elsewhere in Asia.[3]

Eating disorders have higher rates among college students. Anorexia affects 0.6% to 2% of college women and 0.2% to 1.1% of college men; bulimia rates in college are 3% to 14% for women and 0.02% to 0.2% for men.[4] Some studies suggest higher rates among athletes and comparable rates among military cadets as among civilian students. Eating disorder symptoms can morph over time, from a more restrictive underweight anorexic pattern to a binge-purge cycle, or the reverse. Especially in working with college students, the concept of a spectrum of disordered eating is most helpful, since many students exhibit health-threatening behaviors related to food and body image that may not meet full diagnostic criteria for a disorder but nevertheless significantly affect their physical and emotional health and compromise their ability to progress through college. More and more, it's clear that early intervention can prevent chronicity.

Assessment Considerations

In the vignette above, Nicole's presentation initially suggests a variety of possible diagnoses, ranging from unrecognized ADHD to depression, dysthymia, anxiety or panic, or a nonpsychiatric problem (dehydration, a thyroid abnormality, a viral illness). Without screening, the eating symptoms might not have surfaced. She is defensive and dismissive about the possible contribution of disordered eating to her current problem. It's important to be sensitive to her reluctance to address eating concerns, while still being thorough in assessing for an eating disorder. Eating disorders frequently co-occur with depression, anxiety, and addictions, with comorbidity rates ranging from 23% to as high as 90%.[5] Missing an eating disorder diagnosis and thus failing to address the disorder makes it extremely unlikely that the comorbid condition will significantly improve.

In a random sample of nearly 3,000 students at a large midwestern university, researchers screened for eating disorders using the SCOFF questionnaire (a five-item screen shown to be effective in university samples), finding that 13.5% of females and 3.5% of males screened positive and that the majority of these students had never gotten treatment.[6] When these students were followed for two years, symptoms persisted in more than half, and again, many never got treatment. Comorbidity rates in this sample were also high. Many of the students who screened positive did perceive a need for help, but most did not seek mental health treatment. This underscores the importance of screening for disordered eating, and the SCOFF questions can be easily inserted either as a written screen into a student's initial paperwork, or orally into an intake interview (see table 12.1). A "yes" on two or more items strongly suggests an eating disorder; three "yes" answers increases the likelihood of an eating disorder by elevenfold.[7]

Nicole's reticence to discuss her disordered eating might shift our focus to her anxiety symptoms and academic distress, at least initially. Further questions

Table 12.1   SCOFF screening questions

Do you ever make yourself sick because you feel uncomfortably full?
Do you worry you may have lost control over how much you eat?
Have you recently lost more than 14 pounds ("one stone") in a three-month period?
Do you believe yourself to be fat when others say you are too thin?
Would you say that food dominates your life?

to assess eating and body image, including those in table 12.1, are best asked in the context of gathering general health information. If a student is particularly reluctant to answer questions about her eating habits, I provide psychoeducation within the assessment portion of the session, saying something like, "Sometimes people turn to food to control powerful emotions, and it's their best effort at remaining emotionally in control. When people develop an eating disorder, the symptoms actually at first help them cope with another problem that has overwhelmed them; we don't ask them to give up the symptom until they have developed healthier ways to cope with whatever else was causing them such distress." I also stress the physiological links between eating and proper hydration and concentration, dizziness, and energy to help the student begin to acknowledge those connections.

In all students with body image concerns, but especially in those who appear obviously underweight, or who report patterns of significant restriction, a clear understanding of exactly what and how they are eating is crucial. This includes finding out how many calories a day they consume as well as whether they have "safe" or "good" foods and "unsafe" or "bad" foods, consider themselves under- or overweight, feel a loss of control over eating, and continue to have a menstrual period. Many college women take oral contraceptives, which can mask amenorrhea. Since the amenorrhea criterion has been eliminated from DSM-5, its presence is no longer relevant to diagnosis but still gives us important information about a woman's health.

Nicole endorses multiple symptoms of depression over the past two months, many beginning when a boyfriend who'd once commented negatively on her weight broke up with her. She'd started midnight ice cream runs with her roommate in an attempt to feel better, but this led to binging, then feeling disgusted with herself afterward, followed by marathon sessions at the gym, where she spent two to three hours exercising to get rid of the extra calories. In the past two weeks, she's organized much of her time around being able to get to the gym almost daily. She's lost about five pounds and received compliments from several friends. She sees this as "getting healthy again" but is perplexed about experiencing dizziness after and sometimes during exercise. Although she denies dieting excessively, she admits that sometimes she skips meals to "save" her calories for going out drinking with friends in the evening.

In fact, she had been out drinking the night before the exam that prompted her referral. Prior to that, she'd never had panic symptoms. She has been increasingly alarmed by her declining academic performance, had slept poorly before the exam, and had felt unprepared. During the exam, she repeatedly berated herself for being irresponsible and drinking, and she imagined failing out of college and having to tell her parents. She had passive suicidal ideation (without plan or intent) during the exam, and admits this has also occurred at other times over the past month.

Nicole has never made a suicide attempt, but admits that on occasion she cuts herself. This began in middle school, when she was somewhat pudgy and socially isolated. She slimmed down when she ran track in high school and has refrained from any cutting the past two years after a previous boyfriend was very disturbed by the behavior. However, in the past two months the urge to cut has intensified. She has multiple superficial healing lacerations on her forearm. She has never received mental health treatment before, though she's thought about it. Her mother has been treated for depression, and her father "drinks too much." Her mother is diabetic and obese and has been advised to lose weight.

Nicole's symptoms suggest a diagnosis of a depressive disorder. Her disordered eating symptoms don't meet duration criteria for bulimia nervosa, but they do suggest another specified eating disorder diagnosis, in DSM-5 terms, that could, if symptoms continue, develop into full-blown bulimia. Although many college students—and clinicians!—associate the term "purging" with self-induced vomiting, college students more commonly try to control weight via other compensatory behaviors, such as excessive exercise or fasting.[8] Because exercise has so many health benefits, it often takes longer for both students and clinicians to recognize when exercise has become problematic unless intentionally screening for it. Similarly, many students are preoccupied with eating more healthfully, but when this becomes extreme, it may also be part of an eating disorder. Termed "orthorexia," this rigid insistence on eliminating fats or skewing the diet in a health-threatening direction must also be addressed if present.

Bulimia more often than anorexia first presents in college. Binging, purging, and alcohol abuse also commonly co-occur, so the ubiquity of alcohol use on campus may be one contributing factor to the rise of bulimia in this setting.[9] It's also possible that similar personality traits, mood states, or impulsivity contribute to both types of binge behaviors. Eating disorders in general have high rates of genetic heritability, with about a third of risk for the eating disorder, depression, anxiety, or addiction being shared.[10] Regardless, the confluence of binge eating and binge drinking can have significant consequences. "Saving calories" for alcohol is a concerning finding in Nicole's presentation, and her evaluation must include a thorough review of substance use. Studies suggest that more severe dieting and binging is more strongly associated not with prevalence of alcohol use per se, but with more frequent intoxication and more negative consequences, such as blackouts or unwanted sexual encounters.[11] College women who both binge eat and binge drink are five times as likely to report problems at work or school, three times as likely to have problems with friends, and three times as likely to have been involved in a sexual situation they regretted.[12]

Nicole is also engaging in non-suicidal self-injury (NSSI), which frequently occurs along with eating disorder symptoms and with substance abuse. Although NSSI was long considered a cardinal symptom of borderline personality disorder, it's increasingly clear that it can accompany a variety of psychological problems and is not rare among college students. In a random sample of more than 2,800 undergraduate and graduate students at two northeastern universities, lifetime prevalence of at least one incident of self-injurious behavior (without suicidal intent) was 17%; over 70% of that group engaged in multiple incidents.[13] In this sample, those with NSSI were more likely to be female, be bisexual or questioning, have a history of emotional or sexual abuse, and have at least one symptom of an eating disorder or other indicators of increased psychological distress. NSSI also occurs more frequently in people whose suicide risk is elevated, but usually, as also described in the DSM-5, the person engages in NSSI to bring about relief from intense negative feelings, to resolve interpersonal difficulties, or to experience "release," or positive emotions, rather than to end her life. Maternal depression, non-heterosexual orientation, affective dysregulation, and depression were independent predictors of past-year NSSI in another large longitudinal study of college students and self-injury, which also found that coping, mental distress, and situational stressors were common motives[14] for the behavior. In this study, one in six with NSSI attempted suicide by young adulthood, so although it's important not to overreact to all cutting or other self-harm incidents, it's always good practice to do a thorough risk assessment when these are present. NSSI occurs in many students without eating issues, it's possible that some of the same neurobiological factors that underlie the emotional reactivity and impulsivity that lead to cutting also underlie binging and purging behaviors.

Binge eating without concurrent compensatory behaviors is an even more common complaint among college students. Binge eating disorder has been added to the roster of feeding and eating disorders in the DSM-5 to describe individuals who experience loss of control over episodes of excessive eating that occur at least weekly for three months and cause significant psychological and physical distress.[15] Binge eating affects more males and more women of color than other forms of disordered eating, and it is strongly correlated with depression, binge drinking, diabetes, and other health problems.[16] Because this form of disordered eating responds to psychiatric treatment, recognizing its presence among university students and addressing it will likely improve life for a broad range of students.

Patterns of Disordered Eating in Men and Other "Nontraditional" Groups

Although men make up a minority of eating disorder patients in community clinical samples—often less than 10%—they are increasingly expressing disordered eating behaviors or body image concerns in college samples. Gay and bisexual college men are one group at greater risk for eating disorders, scoring higher on the Eating Disorders Inventory (EDI-2) than straight men and scoring especially high on drive for thinness, body dissatisfaction, and body image–related anxiety.[17] Like women with eating disorders, men with eating disorders have much higher rates of other psychiatric illnesses. Even among straight men, body image dissatisfaction appears to be on the rise, especially in men who want a more muscular body type and engage in restrictive eating or compulsive exercising behaviors to try to bulk up.[18] And in certain parts of the country, eating disordered behaviors are on the rise among adolescent boys. A recent survey by the CDC and the Los Angeles Unified School District found that high school boys in LA are twice as likely as boys nationwide to purge or use laxatives, and as likely as girls to use diet pills without medical advice.[19] Steroid use is also increasingly common among teenage boys, in part to sculpt muscles to media-portrayed ideals but also to enhance athletic performance. As the next cohorts of boys enter college, we may see further increases in body image concerns among college men.

Some studies have suggested that lesbian and bisexual women have lower rates of eating disorders compared with heterosexual women, but more recent studies find the rates are comparable.[20] In this group, as in others, the high level of comorbidity between eating disorders and depression, anxiety, and substance abuse underscore the importance of remaining alert to the possibility of disordered eating. Some studies suggest that clinicians may screen less often in groups they consider less likely to have an eating disorder, such as students from ethnic minority backgrounds. In part this may be because of reports that, for example, African American women have much lower rates of anorexia than Caucasian women. But might this be due to disparities in the way different people access health care services, or to other confounding demographic variables, such as socioeconomic status, more than ethnicity?

A recent study of college students involved in an eating disorders screening program across several universities found that the frequency of four eating disorder symptoms and two exercise symptoms did not differ among women from Caucasian, African American, Asian American/Pacific Islander, Latino, or Native American/Alaskan Native backgrounds.[21] The researchers did find some differences in compensatory behaviors by ethnicity. For example, Asian Americans were less likely to use diuretics, and Native Americans were more likely to use laxatives and multiple methods of purging. Types of distress reported by students of different ethnicities also varied: Caucasian, African American and Latino students found binge eating to be the most upsetting symptom assessed, while Asian American students were most distressed by vomiting. Asian women who report laxative use are less likely to be referred for eating disorder evaluation or treatment than Caucasian women. Thus bias in the clinician's index of suspicion for an eating disorder as well as in the student's tendency to seek treatment depending on cultural background and other factors, may conspire to make us miss disordered eating in some groups.

It's not entirely clear whether eating disorder symptoms remain stable within individuals throughout college. Some studies find increases over time, and others decreases. However, several longitudinal studies agree on risk factors for eating disorders in these students: depression, body dissatisfaction, low self-esteem, body weight outside of healthy parameters, and stress.[22] Nicole has several of these risk factors, but she does not have a history of an eating disorder and has been binging and exercising excessively for only a couple of months. These are good prognostic factors. Early intervention is critical to preventing chronicity in eating disorders, and sharing this fact with students can help motivate them for treatment.

Table 12.2   Recommended laboratory tests in patients who have eating disorders

All eating disorder patients	Malnourished or severely symptomatic	Amenorrhea for more than 6 months	Frequent binging/purging
CBC with differential	Complement component 3	Osteopenia and osteoporosis assessments	Serum amylase
Serum electrolytes, BUN, creatinine			
TSH, or thyroid profile	Ca, Mg, P, Ferritin		Urine toxicology screen
Erythrocyte sed rate	EKG		Beta-HCG
AST/ALT, alkaline phosphatase	24-hour urine for creatinine clearance		
Urinalysis			

Source: Adapted from American Psychiatric Association. (2006). *Practice guideline for the treatment of patients with eating disorders* (3rd ed.). Arlington, VA: American Psychiatric Association.

Sometimes, understanding the link between disordered eating and depression or anxiety will also help a student overcome her reluctance to get the full assessment that is ideally part of every disordered eating work-up. This would include referral to a nutritionist who is skilled in working with eating disorder clients, a physical exam and bloodwork when indicated, and usually, completion of the EDI-2. This well-validated instrument measures both risk and symptoms of eating disorders, in college men as well as women.[23] The EDI-2 can be particularly helpful in determining not only the diagnosis but also the appropriate level of care to best treat the student (more on levels of care in the treatment section below.)

Nicole's presentation illustrates mild to moderate disordered eating symptoms of short duration, the more common constellation among college students. A significant number of students, however, do present with significant anorexia or bulimia. Some of these students have already had extensive treatment before or during college. In these cases, baseline laboratory work and a physical exam is critical and, according to American Psychiatric Association practice guidelines, should include the tests listed in table 12.2.

Vital in the assessment of a student with an eating disorder is evaluating her medical stability and determining the appropriate level of care.

Treatment Considerations

Eating disorders and disordered eating in general require a true bio-psycho-social approach, best accomplished through collaboration among psychiatrists, primary care doctors, therapists, nutritionists, and at times, dentists. For adolescents, family involvement in treatment is also very important: APA practice guidelines and those of other groups, including the UK's National Center for Excellence in Clinical Care (NICE), recommend family therapy based on the Maudsley approach. But what about involving the families of college students?

There's a scant evidence base for best practices in this population. Of course, students who have struggled with an eating disorder for years before college may still be at an early adolescent developmental phase, but they're living on campus and expected to function at a different level. NICE guidelines recommend involving the caretakers of even adult patients with anorexia, and it generally benefits the patient if her family understands how best to help.[24] The level of family participation will be based on the nature of the eating disorder, the age and developmental level of the student, the complexity of the student's needs, and other factors. Certainly when a student is referred to a level of care higher than outpatient, the family must often be involved.

Regardless of how engaged the student's family is, treatment of disordered eating usually requires a team approach. Treatment in a specialized setting or by an outpatient team with experience in treating eating disorders is the ideal, but college students frequently lack access or motivation. As a result, college counseling center psychiatrists, therapists, and student health services physicians are frequently left to do their best to address disordered eating in a suboptimal setting. At Duke we have an interdisciplinary Eating and Body Image Concerns (EBIC) treatment team that meets regularly and reviews all students who signed consent for the team approach as part of their treatment. This helps ensure that the complexities of diagnosis and care are addressed for each student with disordered eating.

APA and NICE practice guidelines are helpful in determining a student's appropriateness for specific levels of care, from outpatient to partial hospital or residential to inpatient hospitalization. Because students may withhold information initially, or the diagnostic picture may change, accurately assessing level of care can take some time. The initial evaluation of a student with disordered eating complaints may take longer to complete than that for other problems. At Duke we've developed an algorithm based on APA guidelines to assess appropriate level of care, and we find it helpful both practically, as we select

Table 12.3   Levels of care for eating disorders

	Level 1*	Level 2	Level 3
Medical complications	Medically stable to the extent that more extensive medical monitoring as defined in levels 4 and 5 is not required	Medically stable to the extent that more extensive medical monitoring as defined in levels 4 and 5 is not required	Medically stable to the extent that more extensive medical monitoring as defined in levels 4 and 5 is not required 3+ Medically stable to the extent that intravenous fluids, nasogastric tube feedings, or multiple daily laboratory tests are not needed
Suicidality	No intent or plan	No intent or plan	No intent or plan 3+ Possible plan but no intent: acute vs. chronic; personal history vs. family history ability to contract
Weight as percentage of healthy body weight**	>85%	>80%	>80%
Motivation to recovery	Fair to good	Fair	Partial; preoccupied with ego-syntonic thoughts more than 3 hours a day; cooperative
Comorbid disorders (substance abuse, depression, anxiety)	Presence of comorbid condition may influence choice of level of care	Presence of comorbid condition may influence choice of level of care	Presence of comorbid condition may influence choice of level of care
Structure needed for eating and gaining weight	Self-sufficient	Self-sufficient	Needs some structure to gain weight 3+ Needs supervision at all meals or will restrict eating

Level 4	Level 5	Level 6
Medically stable to the extent that intravenous fluids, nasogastric tube feedings, or multiple daily laboratory tests are not needed	*Adults:* HR < 40 bpm; BP < 90/60; glucose < 60 mg/dl; potassium < 3 meq/l; electrolyte imbalance; temp < 97.0° F; dehydration; hepatic, renal, or cardiovascular organ compromise requiring acute treatment *Child/adolescent:* HR in 40s; ortho-static BP changes (>20 bpm increase in HR or >10 to 20 mm Hg drop); BP < 80/50 mm Hg; hypokalemia or hypophosphatemia	—
Possible plan but no intent: acute vs. chronic; personal history vs. family history ability to contract	Intent and plan	—
<85%	<85% (for children and adolescents: acute weight decline with food refusal even if not <85% healthy body weight)	<75% Weight was refractory to levels 1–5 Total parenteral nutrition (TPN)
Fair to poor; preoccupied with ego-syntonic thoughts more than 3 hours a day; cooperative with highly structured treatment	Poor to very poor; preoccupied with ego-syntonic thoughts 4–6 hours a day; uncooperative with treatment or cooperative only in highly structured environment	—
Presence of comorbid condition may influence choice of level of care	Any existing psychiatric disorder that would require hospitalization	
Needs supervision at all meals or will restrict eating	Needs supervision during and after meals or nasogastric/special feeding	Needs medical supervision or refusing oral feeding but amenable to TPN

Continued

Table 12.3   (continued)

	Level 1*	Level 2	Level 3
Impairment and ability to care for self; ability to control exercise	Able to exercise for fitness and control compulsive exercising	Able to exercise for fitness and control compulsive exercising	Structure required to prevent patient from compulsive exercise
Purging behavior (laxatives and diuretics)	Can greatly reduce purging in unstructured settings; no significant medical complications such as ECG abnormalities that would suggest the need for hospitalization	Can greatly reduce purging in unstructured settings; no significant medical complications such as ECG abnormalities that would suggest the need for hospitalization	Can greatly reduce purging in unstructured settings; no significant medical complications such as ECG abnormalities that would suggest the need for hospitalization
Environmental stress	Others able to provide adequate emotional and practical support and structure	Others able to provide adequate emotional and practical support and structure	Others able to provide at least limited support and structure
			3+ (>18) Severe family conflict, problems, or absence so that family unable to provide structured treatment in home, or lives alone without adequate support system

Source: Adapted from American Psychiatric Association. (2006). *Practice guideline for the treatment of patients with eating disorders* (3rd ed.). Arlington, VA: American Psychiatric Association.

Level 1: outpatient. *Level 2:* intensive outpatient. *Level 3:* day hospital or partial hospitalization. *Level 3+:* hybrid PHP (7 days a week, 11 hours per day with alternative living situation). *Level 4:* residential treatment center. *Level 5:* inpatient hospitalization. *Level 6:* acute medical ICU and step down.

**The rule of thumb for healthy body weight is as follows. *Men:* 106 lbs. for the first 5 ft. and 6 lbs. per inch thereafter (BMI = 23.8). *Women:* 100 lbs. for the first 5 ft. and 5 lbs. per inch thereafter (BMI = 21).

Level 4	Level 5	Level 6
Complete role impairment; cannot eat and gain weight by self; structure required to prevent patient from compulsive exercising	Complete role impairment; cannot eat and gain weight by self; structure required to prevent patient from compulsive exercising	Complete role impairment; cannot eat and gain weight by self; structure required to prevent patient from compulsive exercising
May need supervision during and after all meals and in bathroom	Needs supervision during and after all meals and in bathroom	—
Severe family conflict, problems, or absence so that family unable to provide structured treatment in home, or lives alone without adequate support system	Severe family conflict, problems, or absence so that family unable to provide structured treatment in home, or lives alone without adequate support system	—

treatment, and therapeutically, as we explain to students why we're making a particular recommendation.

Outpatient treatment is a good starting place for Nicole since she's medically stable and her symptoms are relatively new. Both pharmacotherapy with serotonin-reuptake inhibitors and cognitive behavioral therapy are effective treatments for bulimia and are backed by the strongest evidence base, though interpersonal and other behavioral therapies also can be helpful.[25] Although Nicole doesn't meet the full criteria, there is enough in her presentation to suggest she'd benefit from an SSRI and CBT. Dialectical behavior therapy has the best evidence base for reducing NSSI and can also be a great treatment for eating disorder symptoms. At the very least, Nicole's depression should improve with antidepressant treatment, and this may help motivate her to work on the disordered eating as well. There's increasing evidence that binge eating also responds to antidepressant treatment. Therapy can also address Nicole's exercising and help her learn to distinguish fitness goals from calorie-expending goals.

College students often make excellent use of bibliotherapy, and there are many outstanding books about recovery from eating disorders. One good resource is the Gürze Books catalog at www.bulimia.com, "Eating Disorders: Resources for Recovery," which lists hundreds of books, including many for special populations, such as athletes.

When students present with anorexia, medication is rarely helpful until weight is restored. In general, the evidence for both antidepressant efficacy and for psychotherapies other than the Maudsley approach is considered weak in the acute phase of treatment.[26] Many of the psychological symptoms, including the obsessive preoccupation with food and calories, the depressive symptoms, the anxiety, and the cognitive impairment improve with nutritional restoration, though of course the student's extreme reluctance to restore weight and fear of getting fat are the obstacles to this. If a restricting student is sufficiently stable to meet criteria for outpatient care, sometimes an antidepressant or a second-generation antipsychotic such as olanzapine or risperidone can help.[27] In attempting outpatient treatment, it's critical to monitor whether the student is making any progress toward weight restoration. Lack of progress, or stalled progress, requires rapid referral to a higher level of care.

Eating disorders are tenacious and can cause hopelessness in both patients and in those treating them. According to eating disorder specialist Craig Johnson, however, evidence increasingly shows that the probability of recovery goes up with cognitive maturation. This suggests that an emerging adult who has battled disordered eating since her teens may finally have the neurobiological capacity to make good use of treatment during the college or grad school years. It's important to share this perspective with students who have struggled for a long time.

Treatment Challenges

Often, the results of blood tests and the physical exam in a young, otherwise healthy college student may be mostly normal, even when other parts of the assessment suggest a serious eating disorder that requires a higher level of care than outpatient treatment. Normal results can reinforce a student's opinion that nothing is seriously wrong with her. It's important to help her understand that the physical work-up is only one part of the diagnostic picture. If other parts of the assessment suggest a need for a higher level of care—if the student's body weight is hovering near 85% of ideal, with rapid weight loss or perhaps a failure to gain or maintain weight in the outpatient setting—the decision regarding level of care might be made before the test results come back. Significantly abnormal results might then direct a student toward inpatient rather than residential care, but relatively normal results should not then suggest that outpatient care continues to be appropriate if this is contrary to the rest of the assessment.

Students sometimes want to address their eating disorders, but more often they'd prefer to leave that unexamined and instead focus on their presenting concerns of mood or anxiety problems, or on interpersonal difficulties. This presents an ethical dilemma, since untreated eating disorders have the highest lethality of the psychiatric disorders and since, in my experience—and as reflected in a growing body of evidence—not addressing the eating disorder makes it unlikely that the other concerns will significantly improve. However, if the eating disorder is fairly new or less severe—for example, limited to binge eating and rare (less than once a week) purging or other compensatory behavior—then focusing initially on the mood or anxiety component might be a reasonable approach, both to establish a treatment alliance and to build hope. Transparency is important with this approach, letting the student know that we're starting with this particular focus, but we will return to the disordered eating and try other treatment strategies if that does not start to also improve as the other issues improve.

At times, a student who is dangerously underweight, or who is binging and vomiting daily, may minimally engage in outpatient treatment while steadfastly refusing to pursue recommended higher levels of care. In these situations, consultation with colleagues is critical. Often these students have also come to the attention of others on campus, such as concerned peers, professors, or administrators. If it is medically dangerous for that student to continue her semester, collaboration with other campus professionals, within the limits permitted by confidentiality, can help create a plan to put the student on medical leave. In rare instances, medical risk requires that we sacrifice confidentiality. Some universities have developed administrative policies for students with anorexia that require weekly weigh-ins to verify that they are maintaining a target weight in order to continue in school. This requires us to balance a student's civil rights with health and safety, but it also demonstrates to students the reality that unless they tend to their health, it is unlikely that they will be able to make much of the opportunities college—or life—affords them.

CHAPTER 13

Difficulty Concentrating

University life challenges students in many ways: intellectually, emotionally, physically, and socially. But almost all students see their primary goals on campus as academic, so problems that interfere with their concentration and academic performance rapidly get their attention and send them seeking help. Given the explosion of distractions on campus, especially with the advent of the digital age and social media, students increasingly complain of trouble concentrating. Sorting out the main culprit, and then finding remedies, is often complicated by many confounding factors.

Tom, a 19-year-old biracial gay male planning to major in engineering, has found it more and more difficult to focus on schoolwork since the beginning of his sophomore year. He performed well academically freshman year, but half his classes were familiar to him from his advanced placement classes in high school. This year he's easily bored, doesn't enjoy his classes, and zones out in lectures. His mind wanders when he studies for more than an hour, and he forgets what he's just read. He borrowed his fraternity brother's Ritalin twice this past week and felt more focused, awake, and able to study longer. He thinks he may have undiagnosed attention-deficit hyperactivity disorder (ADHD). He was an excellent student up through high school, but as the only child in his family, he benefitted from his Korean-born father's constant attention to his schoolwork and frequent homework help. His father also devised additional assignments for Tom in math, so he'd be ahead. His Caucasian, Californian mother has encouraged him to be "more relaxed." Tom denies symptoms of depression and general anxiety, other than anxiety about poor academic performance. He is out to friends in college but not to his family or friends back home.

Diversion of stimulants to students for whom they have not been prescribed, or nonmedical stimulant use, has grown and become more socially acceptable among college students. More children with ADHD are treated in high school and thus can go to college, increasing the availability of stimulants on campus. Rates of nonmedical use vary across the country, ranging from 0% to 25% in student populations, with an average rate of 8%; higher rates are typically seen at more selective, competitive universities.[1] Like Tom, most students have access to stimulants via other students, who share or sell their medication. The most common reason for nonmedical stimulant use is to improve concentration, with the goal of improving academic performance; although some of these students also use stimulants recreationally, a small minority of nonmedical users take these drugs solely to get high or for other nonacademic reasons.[2] But stimulants improve concentration in most people, so this fact alone doesn't make a diagnostic case for ADHD for Tom.

ADHD is a disorder with childhood onset, but not all cases are diagnosed in childhood, and symptoms change through adolescence into adulthood. Hyperactivity symptoms tend to be less prominent by college, and although the hyperactive subtype remains the most common diagnostically, in the college setting inattentive symptoms cause the greatest impairment. So most students using nonprescribed stimulants probably don't have ADHD, but a minority of them might. ADHD affects between 4% and 8% of college students, and in contrast to the childhood gender disparity (boys outnumber girls nearly 4 to 1), the gender distribution is more equal in college.[3]

Using a validated symptom checklist that was adapted for college students, one large study at two southern universities found that students with more self-reported inattentive symptoms had higher nonmedical stimulant use even after controlling for many other factors, including use of other prescription drugs, depressive symptoms, or other substance abuse.[4] Depressive symptoms actually decreased the odds that a student would use a stimulant. Students who had many hyperactivity and impulsivity symptoms, however, were more likely to use other prescription drugs and to abuse substances. The authors concluded that although students who use stimulants for which they don't have a prescription are concentrated within the groups of students prone to substance abuse, the majority of them are in fact using stimulants because they struggle academically due to inattentive symptoms.

As more research focuses on college students with ADHD, certain characteristics emerge. These students have lower GPAs, are more likely to be on academic probation or fail to complete college, and work longer and harder than peers without ADHD.[5] They tend to use substances more, including earlier and more frequent use of tobacco and marijuana, and they suffer greater negative consequences of problematic alcohol use.[6] However, they may also have unique resilience. Although large epidemiological studies of adults and children with ADHD find much higher rates of depression and anxiety disorders than among people without the condition, one recent study that compared college students with ADHD to students without found no differences in depressive or anxiety symptoms, as measured by the Beck Depression and Anxiety inventories; the few other existing studies on college students have not consistently found differences.[7]

ADHD rates vary among different ethnic groups and between international students and American students, but the data are somewhat inconsistent. One study, for example, found that more African Americans than white students suffered from ADHD symptoms as assessed by a self-report measure (8.4% versus 2.3%), but that when parents were asked to retrospectively report symptoms, the ratio flipped, with more white than African American students meeting criteria.[8]

Depression, anxiety, psychotic disorders, and substance abuse all impair concentration, and it's important to rule those out—or treat comorbid conditions, which are common in people with ADHD—when considering a diagnosis of ADHD in a previously undiagnosed college student. Academic difficulties are also a predictor of suicide in college students, and since suicide risk is greater among LGBT students, a careful risk assessment is vital for a student like Tom. Other stressors, such as Tom remaining closeted to his family, may be a distraction, but he denies significant emotional fallout from this issue, nor did it seem to cause problems for him in his freshman year. It's also important to ask Tom about his interest in his chosen field of study, given his father's insistence on acceleration in math when Tom was in high school. Sometimes boredom or flagging concentration suggests that a student is pursuing coursework to please someone else.

Assuming Tom does not have a comorbid psychiatric diagnosis, what are the next steps in evaluating his concentration difficulties?

In the age of helicopter parenting, many students arrive at college having had an enormous amount of daily support for academic work, through direct parental help with homework, parental organization and reminders that allowed students to stay organized, or tutoring. The high school day is much more structured than the college day. Some high school environments aren't particularly challenging for bright kids, even kids with attention difficulties. The increased academic demands of college, combined with the lack of supervision, structure, and family support as well as numerous social outlets that compete for students' time all serve to unmask undiagnosed attention difficulties or to exacerbate existing problems. Ironically, although many students without a diagnosis of ADHD use their friends' stimulants to get an academic edge, many students *with* well-documented ADHD diagnoses choose the transition to college as the time to go off their medication, hoping they no longer need it or sometimes feeling as if they're cheating by taking medicine to help with academics. Not surprisingly, these students can have an especially difficult adjustment to college.

ADHD diagnoses account for about half of the accommodations granted to college students.[9] Some students who struggle academically might see an ADHD diagnosis as a route to accommodations or stimulants, so a careful evaluation must not rely exclusively on symptom self-report. Because of the chronic nature of the disorder, some college counseling centers, including Duke's, refer out those students with an existing diagnosis as well as students who screen positive and need diagnostic evaluation. But assuming that's not possible, what's the best way to evaluate a college student for ADHD?

Diagnosing ADHD in College or Graduate Students

Current diagnostic categories and symptom descriptions may not be entirely appropriate for emerging adults who have already made it to a university setting. This group may be more mildly affected (having already made it to higher education) or have other skills, abilities, and support networks that allow them to be successful in a postsecondary setting; yet compared with their peers, they may still suffer from a treatable obstacle to reaching their full potential. Many researchers are working on developing better screening tools for this popula-

<u>Instructions:</u> Ask patient to complete this questionnaire. If he/she places an "X" in four or more darkly-shaded boxes, this is a positive screen and further evaluation is warranted.

Patient Name			Today's Date					
Please answer the questions below, rating yourself on each of the criteria shown using the scale on the right side of the page. As you answer each question, place an X in the box that best describes how you have felt and conducted yourself over the past 6 months. Please give this completed checklist to your healthcare professional to discuss during today's appointment.				Never	Rarely	Sometimes	Often	Very Often
1. How often do you have trouble wrapping up the final details of a project, once the challenging parts have been done?						▓	▓	▓
2. How often do you have difficulty getting things in order when you have to do a task that requires organization?						▓	▓	▓
3. How often do you have problems remembering appointments or obligations?						▓	▓	▓
4. When you have a task that requires a lot of thought, how often do you avoid or delay getting started?							▓	▓
5. How often do you fidget or squirm with your hands or feet when you have to sit down for a long time?							▓	▓
6. How often do you feel overly active and compelled to do things, like you were driven by a motor?							▓	▓

Figure 13.1. The Adult ADHD Self-Report Scale (ASRS) Six Question Screener. © World Health Organization.

tion. In the meantime, a good starting point in evaluating students like Tom is the Adult ADHD Self-Report Screener (ASRS), a validated and reliable six-question instrument, developed in conjunction with the World Health Organization, whose sensitivity of 68.7% and specificity of 99.5%[10] make it an excellent brief screen (see figure 13.1). One study of more than 1,000 first-year students at one university compared students with and without ADHD diagnoses on the 18-item version of the ASRS and found that although most students without a diagnosis scored in the low range, about 10% actually did fall into the clinical range.[11] Since the six-item version of the screen appears to be as effective as the longer version, however, it's more convenient to use the shorter version.

If the student screens positive, the following next steps[12] are useful:

1. Assess frequency and severity of symptoms in the past six months, using both symptom scales—including full version of ASRS, or another

measure, such as the College ADHD Response Evaluation (CARE) scale, a 90-item self-report and 44-item parent report inventory that can also identify areas to target in treatment—and the clinical interview. The Connors Continuous Performance Test (C-CPT) is a direct assessment measure that is also being studied in college students. The Indiana University Health Center, for example, uses a screening packet comprising the Conner Adult ADD form, to be completed by a parent or guardian; the Wender Utah ADD measure; the Beck Depression Inventory; the Beck Anxiety Inventory; and the Learning and Study Skills Inventory (LASSI). Students are asked to send in their elementary, middle, and high school transcripts and records as well.

2. Evaluate symptom impact on multiple areas, including academic functioning, via interview and outside corroboration: parent, peer, professor, dean report, and academic or work records.

3. Establish childhood history of inattentive or hyperactive symptoms by using school records, parent corroboration if possible, and retrospective symptom rating scales.

4. Take a complete individual and family history, with special consideration of psychiatric comorbidities as described above. Remember to do a substance use assessment.

5. Consider neuropsychological testing.

6. Consider referral for medical work-up if indicated.

In evaluating students with concentration difficulties, it's important to do a full substance use assessment, because heavy alcohol or drug use might easily account for the concentration problem. College students who use marijuana on a near-daily basis show significant deficiencies on neuropsychological testing in attentional/executive functioning, including decreased mental flexibility, increased perseveration, and reduced learning compared to "light" users, even after a day or more of abstinence[13] (see also chapter 7). Among students with ADHD who also misuse stimulant medications, 94% also smoke marijuana, and over a third use it daily.[14] However, these students tend to underestimate or minimize the effects of the substance use.

Tom reports occasional (less than once a month) marijuana use, and drinks "about as much as everyone else in my fraternity"—three to six drinks, two to three nights of the week. He doesn't use tobacco or other drugs. He takes no other prescription medications.

Although ADHD has high comorbidity with substance abuse, studies show that college students with ADHD don't drink more alcohol than their peers without the disorder; they do keep up, however, drinking as much, and they seem more vulnerable to alcohol dependence and other negative consequences of heavy drinking, including doing something they later regret, having a hangover, or being injured.[15] So, although Tom's drinking may be within the "normal" range within his fraternity, if he's ultimately diagnosed with ADHD, he needs to understand that alcohol may cause *him* more problems than it does his brothers.

Treatment Considerations

Students with concentration difficulties who have depression or anxiety should first be treated for those problems, since focus and attention often improve as the other conditions do. In fact, if in treating other conditions, most symptoms remit except for concentration, attention, and organizational problems, ADHD may be the culprit—but only if impairment occurs in at least two areas of the student's life. Simply not doing well in school is not sufficient to make the diagnosis.

Substance abuse, if present, should likewise be a primary target of treatment. Moderate to severe substance use disorders require referral for specialized treatment, and obviously, heavy drug users might first require detoxification. But much more common is to see occasional or intermittent substance use in college students with ADHD. There's controversy in the literature over whether to insist on at least a short period of abstinence before making a diagnosis, or to treat if diagnosis seems likely based on retrospective recall (and parental corroboration) of early symptoms that predated substance use. Many clinicians these days advocate for addressing the substance use, but not withholding ADHD treatment in occasional users.[16] Thus, we'd educate Tom about the effects of alcohol and marijuana on his symptoms, use motivational interviewing to encourage decreased use or abstinence, but also treat for ADHD *if* his *full* evaluation suggests this diagnosis. In students with a recent (within past three months) substance abuse history, medicines with a lower addiction potential are better first choices: atomoxetine, bupropion, or extended-release methylphenidate. Many psychiatrists will not prescribe stimulants in students who continue to use drugs and will use drug testing to enforce treatment contracts.

Some students don't meet criteria for either ADHD or another psychiatric condition; they simply have never developed study habits that are adequate for the level of work required in college and beyond. These students may need academic skills coaching, if that's available on campus. Workshop-style group programs can be effective in addressing issues around stress management, procrastination, and other academic challenges that are common in college. Mindfulness meditation likewise trains students to focus on the present moment and can enhance concentration skills.

If a student does actually have ADHD, however, either newly diagnosed or long standing but still causing problems, treatment usually consists of a combination of psychopharmacology and counseling. Because of the characteristics of the college community, though, with its booming market for stimulant drugs, especially if this is the first time the student has had to manage his medication, prescribing stimulants to college students requires additional vigilance about misuse. Students who begin stimulants in college are more likely to misuse and divert the medication, as are those in fraternities, white students, and those in the northeastern part of the country.[17]

Tom, and students like him, should be educated about *why* it is not a good idea to take someone else's prescribed medication. Students are frequently unaware that it is a criminal offense, and they may not know about the numerous potential side effects of stimulant medications. Some see no problem with "academic doping" as a way to boost GPA, and even the scientific community has raised for discussion the concept of "responsible use of cognitive-enhancing drugs."[18] But of course these medications can have serious physiological effects, ranging from appetite suppression, irritability, and insomnia to cardiac arrhythmias. They can exacerbate anxiety or trigger mania in susceptible individuals. In fact, many psychiatrists routinely screen for worsened anxiety after first prescribing a stimulant. And furthermore, they can be highly addictive.

The *New York Times* recently featured a profile of a pre-med student who became addicted to Adderall and ultimately committed suicide when a doctor finally limited his access to the medication.[19] In this case, the family questioned the diagnosis of ADHD, given the student's lack of any childhood symptoms and that academic difficulties began around the time he started studying for the medical school entrance exams. In my opinion it's good practice to require testing for any emerging adult in whom we are considering a new ADHD diagnosis, but some college psychiatrists have observed that even the testing itself is prone to interpretation bias toward diagnosing ADHD. Self-report measures and performance tests can be subject to symptom exaggeration and negative response bias. Testing is also both expensive and time consuming. Nevertheless, a full diagnostic evaluation with testing might help stem the trend toward more and more students seeking stimulants. As physicians are increasingly pressed for time, there's a real danger that more will prescribe stimulant medicines without a thorough evaluation, and emerging adults, who often demand quick fixes and believe there's a pill for every problem, are particularly likely to press for inappropriate prescribing and especially vulnerable to suffering its consequences.

Some researchers also raise the issue of state-dependent learning, that information assimilated while using a stimulant can only be fully recalled while on the drug again. In the 1970s some papers raised worries about this effect in children treated for ADHD. In 1985, a rigorous study of 40 hyperactive children treated with methylphenidate (which also included a review of existing literature on this topic) found no evidence of state-dependent learning and concluded that their results "did diminish concerns" about this possibility.[20] I could find no studies addressing this in emerging adults; however, animal studies continue to show that retention of certain types of information learned while under the influence of amphetamines *is* state-dependent,[21] and that dose is a significant factor in the types of cognitive effects that amphetamines exert.[22] Students who take diverted stimulants may take any of several amphetamine-type substances, at unclear doses, self-increasing their doses erratically. A discussion of the possibility of state-dependent effects, among the other possible undesired effects, may enable them to more accurately evaluate whether taking stimulants in this way is a risk they're willing to take.

Some college counseling centers that prescribe stimulants have clear guidelines around requirements before these medicines will be prescribed—such as diagnostic testing and documentation of childhood onset of symptoms—and also use a stimulant contract with the student. One such example is the contract used by University Health Services at the University of Wisconsin at Madison (see figure 13.2.) This contract educates the student about the possible risks of this treatment and serves as informed consent for urine drug screens, which can be used to monitor for drugs of abuse if there's clinical suspicion. Based on an informal survey, however, most counseling centers don't seem to routinely incorporate drug testing into their treatment protocols for prescribing stimulants.

Stimulants remain the most commonly used medication class for ADHD among college students. Their use in this population has increased, with the

Stimulant Medication Agreement

To help reach the academic and personal goals I have set, stimulant medication is being prescribed for me. In order to make this medication safe and follow national and state laws, I —

_____ understand that:
      (patient's name)

—This medication may only partially treat my problems.
—I should follow the directions given to me by my prescriber. I will not take more than what I am told.
—Taking alcohol or illegal drugs along with this medication is dangerous.
—My body may get used to the medication and if I stop it too quickly I could feel sick (withdrawal).
—Some people have become addicted to these medications. If I think this is happening to me I will discuss with my prescriber.

Patient's Signature _____ Date _____

I _____ agree:
      (patient's name)

—To obtain stimulants only from the prescriber signed below or his/her designee, and to notify my prescriber immediately if I obtain medication from another provider.
—To give urine samples for drug testing and to bring my pills to be counted whenever asked of me.
—Not to use illegal drugs along with this medication. A positive urine drug screen may result in cancellation of my stimulant prescription and require treatment with a non-stimulant medication.
—Not to sell or give away my medication.
—To keep my medication safe. If it is lost or stolen I understand it will be replaced one time only.
—To keep all my appointments. Missed appointments may result in cancellation of my stimulant prescription.
—That my medication can be stopped at any time, after a discussion with my prescriber.

Patient Signature _____ Date _____

Provider Signature _____ Date _____

_____

Figure 13.2. Stimulant Medication Agreement. Courtesy of Eric Heiligenstein, M.D., University Health Services, University of Wisconsin–Madison.

rate of growth in prescriptions to 20- to 39-year-olds more than doubling in the past four years, greatly outpacing the growth in prescriptions to children and adolescents.[23] Various studies suggest that they are very effective, but until recently, no double-blind, controlled study focused specifically on this population. The first such study, published in 2012, found that the prodrug stimulant lisdexamfetamine dimesylate (LDX) significantly reduced inattention, variability of attention, and hyperactivity and restlessness.[24] In a linear, dose-dependent fashion, it also strongly improved executive functioning, including task management, planning, organization, working memory, and study skills, all crucial for success in college. It had less of an effect on impulsivity and behavior regulation. Other medications with reported efficacy in college populations (but lacking the support of double-blind placebo-controlled trials) include the nonstimulant atomoxetine and antidepressants such as bupropion and the SSRIs.[25]

Unfortunately, most of the evidence regarding psychosocial treatments of college students with ADHD remains qualitative, primarily individual case studies. Academic coaching is growing in popularity, and anecdotally effective, but we need more objective data. Cognitive behavioral therapy with a focus on motivation, goal setting, and time management is likely to be helpful for students with this diagnosis. Some counseling centers that do prescribe stimulants require monthly counseling sessions to teach coping skills, and others require academic skills coaching, as a condition of receiving stimulants.

Students with ADHD who continue to struggle with symptoms may be eligible for accommodations under the Americans with Disabilities Act (ADA). Students can be referred to the university's Office of Disability Services. Accommodations for ADHD are individually tailored, but they may include extended time on exams, a reduced-distraction testing environment, or a note taker.

CHAPTER 14

Anxiety

Anxiety and fear are universal human emotions, with significant adaptive functions in our lives. But surveys of college students suggest that in the past decade or two, more are experiencing problematic anxiety. Nearly half of students in the 2011 National College Health Assessment Survey reported experiencing "overwhelming anxiety" within the past year.[1] Some of these were likely facing developmentally normal or short-lived situational anxiety, but others may have been suffering from an anxiety disorder. Clearly anxiety, or stress, as a presenting concern in counseling centers is on the rise, endorsed by 63% of counseling center patients in 2001, compared with only 36% in 1988.[2] It has become the most commonly cited concern among counseling center clients. Untreated, anxiety can become a chronic, debilitating problem. But most anxiety disorders as well as more self-limited developmental anxieties respond well to treatment, especially in emerging adults, who rapidly grasp the concepts of what causes anxiety and how to most effectively approach rather than avoid the problems it can cause.

Diagnosis: Regular Worry versus a Disorder

Mike is a 24-year-old African American second-year medical student from Seattle who comes in complaining of declining academic performance and concerns about whether he has chosen the right profession. He describes feeling a constant sense of dread about school, racing thoughts, difficulty falling asleep, and frequent stomach disturbances. It's hard to face the day. He can't stop obsessing about whether he should be in medical school or not and often thinks about this question while on hospital rounds, causing him to miss questions that the attending physician directs to him. His mind often goes blank during presentations, and his hands tremble if he's holding notes, making him feel unprepared and embarrassed. He's been told to "relax" by several supervisors and has tried to, but to no avail. He was an excellent student as an undergraduate but has not been able to make honors in any of his medical school courses thus far, and he feels ashamed and demoralized by this. He's most afraid that he will fail to take proper care of his patients and flunk out.

Academic demands occasionally trigger anxiety for most students, but when anxiety is sustained and debilitating, an anxiety disorder may be to blame. Among American adults, anxiety disorders are the most common psychiatric illnesses, with a prevalence rate of 13% to 18%.[3] There's less data on the rate of all anxiety disorders among college students. One study found that in a sample of nearly 3,000 undergraduate and graduate students at a large midwestern university, 4.2% screened positive for either generalized anxiety disorder (GAD) or panic disorder based on the PHQ-9 questionnaire, with GAD being the more common diagnosis.[4] In this study, more women than men suffered from anxiety (mirroring the general population), and more than a third who had anxiety also had some form of depression. One-fifth of those who screened positive for GAD also had suicidal thoughts.

Students frequently use the word "stress" to describe anxiety, though at times it may also refer to depressive symptoms. It's important to get a clear picture of exactly what they mean. Do they feel nervous, tense, afraid, anxious? Is there a sense of physical restlessness or irritability? How long and in what contexts have they been noticing this? Mike also uses the word "obsessing," as students frequently do, but it's helpful to distinguish between occasional irrational worries or constant excessive worries about usual life events, which more typically suggest generalized anxiety, and true obsessive thoughts, which are intrusive, often ego-dystonic, sometimes bizarre or embarrassing, and more commonly accompanied by compulsions. In DSM-5, obsessive-compulsive disorder is separated from the anxiety disorders chapter. Had Mike described a constant thought that he might harm his patients, for example, or intrusive images of actually harming patients, an OCD-spectrum diagnosis may have been more likely.

Other psychiatric conditions can cause or mimic anxiety. The complaint of "racing thoughts" is common among students, and it's important to clarify whether this is an anxiety symptom or a manic or hypomanic one. A newly emerging psychosis can also cause significant anxiety. Anxiety disorders have high rates of comorbidity with other psychiatric problems—especially, for college students, substance abuse.

Mike describes uncertainty over career choice, a developmentally common concern for both graduate and undergraduate students. Probing the specifics of this is important. Did he go to medical school to please family? Did other external or cultural reasons turn him toward a career for which he has little passion? Or is an underlying anxiety problem making him second-guess every decision in his life, thus interfering with his ability to enjoy what perhaps *is* his own chosen path? Would insight-oriented psychotherapy focusing on his hopes and dreams help him untangle this, or is it more appropriate to proceed with cognitive behavioral therapy, more narrowly targeting the anxiety symptoms? And what about medications?

Many of these questions are best addressed through a flexible, creative, and collaborative approach that presents the student with choices for treatment and acknowledges the complexity of his presentation at this time. Diagnostic clarity will also help guide the treatment recommendations. (See figure 14.1 for an algorithm on evaluating anxiety.) Students sometimes present with symptoms across several of the anxiety disorders, without meeting full diagnostic criteria for any one in particular; asking screening questions for all the anxiety disorders should help refine the diagnostic impression. Screening inventories such as the Beck Anxiety Inventory or the Yale-Brown Obsessive-Compulsive Scale can be useful not only in clarifying diagnosis, but also in monitoring treatment response.

> Mike admits he has been a worrier much of his life, though it caused him few problems before in school or in relationships. He denies having been particularly shy and in fact describes himself as "easygoing" prior to medical school.

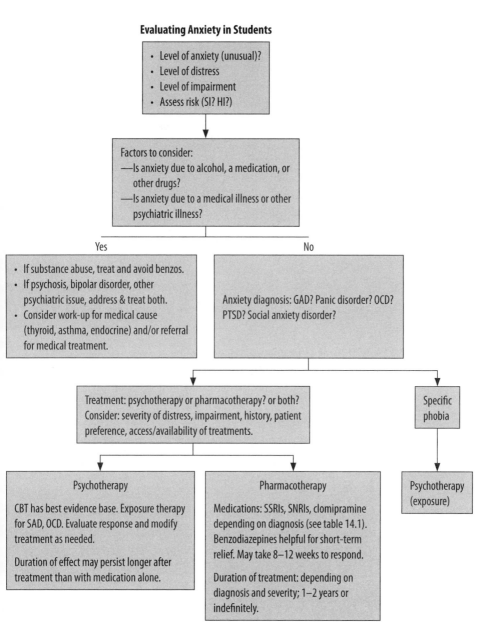

Figure 14.1. Evaluating Anxiety in Students. *Source:* Adapted from American Psychiatric Association Practice Guidelines and Swinson R. P., Antony, M. M., Bleau, P. B., et al. (2006), "Clinical Practice Guidelines: Management of Anxiety *Disorders." Canadian Journal of Psychiatry,* 51 (suppl 2): 1–92.

He found life on the West Coast more laid back and dealt with feelings of restlessness or tension when they occurred by hiking or participating in sports, or by socializing with his friends in Seattle. None of these outlets are as readily available at his East Coast medical school. He did frequently daydream as a child and adolescent but was not hyperactive. Although good at science, he double-majored in philosophy and biology and enjoyed thinking deeply. He finds the amount of material in medical school daunting and the content somewhat boring, and he feels "slow" compared to peers. He was worried and tense through much of his first year of medical school, but all these symptoms abated at home over the summer in Seattle. He denies a trauma history or panic attacks, but in addition to hands shaking and mind going blank during presentations, he has tachycardia and flushing. He denies wanting to harm himself but has been more preoccupied with thoughts of death and feeling like he's not sure there's a point to life.

Generalized Anxiety Disorder and Social Anxiety Disorder

In differentiating developmental anxiety from an anxiety disorder, consider severity and duration of symptoms, context, and impairment. Mike's difficult-to-control worry has been interfering with his academic performance for about 18 months and is intensifying rather than abating. If it were simply a matter of considering his career choice, he might have been able to work through it by now and make a decision, but he worries about several career-related questions and is unable to move forward with any changes. Excessive worry alone is not sufficient to diagnose generalized anxiety disorder (GAD), and in fact studies show that a significant proportion of college students worry excessively but most don't have GAD. One large study that compared undergraduates who were "high worriers" with and without GAD found that the GAD high worriers worried more days than not—more frequently than the non-GAD high worriers—and felt less control over their worry, felt greater impairment specifically due to the worry, and suffered muscle tension and feelings of restlessness significantly more frequently than non-GAD high worriers.[5]

The clinical picture for Mike is most suggestive of generalized anxiety disorder: pervasive worry, muscle tension, sleep difficulties, and mind going blank. DSM-5 reports that GAD is more frequently encountered in adults of European rather than non-European descent, and in women more than men. The literature describes GAD as a chronic condition that persists across contexts, but in my experience working with students, it's not unusual for symptoms to occur at school and then diminish during summers or semesters away from campus. It's almost as if for some people, there's a level of anxiety that simmers just below the diagnostic threshold, and the substantial demands of college or graduate school tip the balance toward the full boil of a clinical problem.

In addition to academic demands, college and graduate or professional school place physical and social demands on emerging adults. Medical school in particular is notorious for interfering with sleep and eating routines. The culture of medicine is one of intense focus on work, with students' mentors frequently modeling poor self-care. We often have to remind students in the healing professions to also take care of their own health, in order to be well enough to care for others.

Anxiety can interfere with working memory, and even students without generalized anxiety often complain of test anxiety or performance anxiety. Again, the need for clinical intervention rests on the severity of impairment. Mike describes several physiological symptoms of performance anxiety that do impair his learning, and that should respond well to treatment. Most likely, anxiety is compromising his academic functioning, but it's also worthwhile to consider whether he might have undiagnosed ADHD. Though it would be unusual for someone to perform so well academically that they're admitted to medical school and still have an undiagnosed learning issue, it's not impossible.

Mike's significant performance anxiety might be considered a variant of social phobia, or social anxiety disorder, nongeneralized subtype, although its absence from earlier periods of his life is intriguing. Is he part of a racial minority group at his medical school, and if so, in what way might this experience affect his confidence and social ease? Some minority students describe the pressure of being the "token" whose performance must stand in for the capabilities of a whole group of people. Even for some nonminority students with an anxious temperament, a poor performance, as the stakes are raised in college or professional school, is so humiliating that they then develop performance anxiety, which abates after treatment, without the need for the more typical ongoing treatment. Had Mike endorsed anxiety in other social situations, he might have been suffering from generalized social anxiety, which afflicts two-thirds of those with social anxiety.[6] Social anxiety disorder is the third most common psychiatric diagnosis in the general population and likely about equally prevalent in campus samples. Interestingly, a study comparing a clinical sample of college students to a nonclinical sample (students taking a psychology class) found similar rates of social phobia based on responses to the Social Phobia Inventory, suggesting that social phobia might be developmentally more common—and thus perhaps not always a disorder—in this population.[7] After all, authors and artists across time have described the social awkwardness and group anxieties of adolescents as they grow into their own areas of comfort with self and peers; these appear quite common in the college years too.

Students with generalized anxiety often have many physical complaints, especially gastrointestinal ones. One large study of undergraduates at UCLA found that of the students who were diagnosed with irritable bowel syndrome (IBS), over 21% also met criteria for GAD, compared with only 7% of students without IBS.[8] Headaches and muscle tension are also frequent complaints. With treatment, many of these symptoms improve along with the psychological symptoms.

Anxiety and Identity

Louise, an 18-year-old Caucasian sophomore from Alabama, comes in complaining of crying spells, fatigue, and loss of interest in cheerleading. She's a member of the college's prestigious cheerleading squad, which guarantees an active social life, but she usually feels like she's just going through the motions and skips social events whenever she can. She was a shy teenager with a very outgoing mother who made sure she was actively involved in the "right kinds" of social activities during high school. She avoids speaking in class, avoids classes that require participation as part of the grade, and suffers significant physiological arousal when she does have to speak up. Cheering isn't hard for her because, she explains, "It's not really me when I'm out there—it's all an act." When asked about friendships and romances, she flushes and says, "And that's another problem. I think I might be bisexual and have a crush on a girl. But I totally don't fit into the whole LGBT scene here, and my family would make me transfer if they knew."

Social anxiety disorder doesn't discriminate—it can affect students who don't, on the surface, appear to be shy or socially isolated. Sometimes it affects the popular fraternity vice president who quells his panic attacks in new social situations with a case of beer, or the pretty cheerleader whom other students see as conformist and popular. Louise illustrates other complexities that arise in diagnosing anxiety in students: she is in the midst of exploring her own sexual orientation and feels unsupported in this in both her family and her campus community. College is a time when students can shed parts of their identity that may not fit them, and this often brings on or exacerbates anxiety. College is also a time when students grapple with existential questions about the meaning of life and their role in the world. Students need clinicians who are open to exploring these questions with them without pathologizing or rushing past them.

For Louise, hiding certain aspects of her identity can account for her anxiety around people she doesn't know well, and the anxiety might abate as she feels more comfortable and can more authentically express herself. However, there's also evidence that the rate of anxiety (and mood) disorders differs according to sexual orientation, with different patterns for men and women. For women who identify as bisexual, the lifetime rates of mood or anxiety disorders are twice as high as for heterosexual women; there are similarly higher rates for bisexual and gay men, but women who are attracted to and have had sex exclusively with women actually have the lowest rates of these psychiatric issues, controlling for other demographic variables.[9]

Emerging adults are also working on other issues of identity formation that can cause anxiety, especially if in conflict with family of origin values and norms. Students may have various other experiences of oppression on campus. Students in racial, ethnic, or religious minority groups may feel isolated or socially awkward due to interacting with people or in situations that differ greatly from what they have previously encountered. International students who were not in a minority group in their home country may suddenly feel intense anxiety accompanying their new experience of being in a minority group on the American campus. It's important to consider these variables in distinguishing "normal" anxiety from the "disorders." At the same time, even students experiencing oppression may have a co-occurring anxiety disorder. A careful patient history, asking if symptoms were ever experienced in the home country or in other home environments; family history; and focus on current impairment can help tease these apart.

Obsessive-Compulsive Spectrum Symptoms

Sometimes, a student who complains of being newly "slower" at completing work than classmates, as Mike did in the vignette above, might be rigidly perfectionistic or procrastinating out of fear of doing poorly. But in some instances this complaint may uncover an obsessive preoccupation with getting things done "just so" or with another intrusive thought that distracts the student. It occasionally can be due to compulsive behaviors or mental rituals, such as the need to count letters in words to have them "even up." Students may misattribute their behavior to being particularly conscientious or thorough, but in some cases their rereading or need to write a perfect sentence prevents them from completing assignments at all, or else causes them to spend untenable amounts of time on simple tasks. Using a scale, such as the Yale-Brown Obsessive-Compulsive Scale (Y-BOCS) can help clarify diagnosis and also monitor treatment efficacy.

According to the National Institute of Mental Health, obsessive-compulsive disorder (OCD) has a lifetime prevalence of about 2% in emerging adults.[10] But among emerging adults in college, higher rates have been reported, especially if we're looking not only at full-criteria OCD but also at the spectrum of symptoms that are fairly common on campus. There's increasing recognition of and interest in obsessive-compulsive-like symptoms and disorders, including body dysmorphic disorder (when an individual is excessively preoccupied with a body part), trichotillomania (hair pulling), pathological skin picking, and health anxiety or hypochondriasis. This group of disorders is now listed in its own category in DSM-5, separately from the anxiety disorders. This is meant to encourage clinicians to also consider the other disorders when one in the cluster seems to be affecting someone. Because OCD has a strong genetic component and because people with OCD have significantly higher rates of other anxiety disorders, some researchers recommended leaving OCD within the anxiety disorders category.[11] Instead, the DSM-5 acknowledges the close relationship between OCD and the other anxiety disorders by listing OCD in the section immediately following the anxiety disorders section.

In my experience, obsessions and compulsions are fairly frequent among college students, and although they don't always rise to the level of a disorder, they cause impairment and thus remain important to assess and address in the course of treatment. A recent study of college students supported this. In a nonclinical volunteer undergraduate sample, some symptoms of an OCD-related disorder were quite common. The authors report that "22% experienced hair pulling urges, and 30% spent at least an hour a day obsessing over a perceived physical flaw or engaged in activities related to this flaw (e.g., staring in the mirror, covering up the flaw)."[12] Perhaps more surprising was that in this sample of students, the rates of symptoms that suggested a full-blown disorder were fairly high. Based on self-report questionnaires, 5% of students met OCD criteria, 5% qualified for a body dysmorphic disorder diagnosis, 3% for trichotillomania, 6% for pathological skin picking, 7% for health anxiety, and these rates were reportedly consistent with rates seen in other studies of college students. Most of the students who qualified for a diagnosis also showed increased overall anxiety compared with students without an OCD-related disorder, and those with pathological skin picking and trichotillomania also had increased impulsivity scores. Thus these are relatively common symptoms in students, and many who experience them are adversely affected but may never seek help.

Panic, Post-traumatic Stress, and Phobias
Occasional unexpected panic attacks are fairly common among college students. In one large nonclinical undergraduate sample, 12% had experienced a panic attack in their lifetime; 2.6% had diagnosable panic disorder.[13] That same study found that although women report more panic attacks, men actually worry more about panic and thus in college samples may be equally at risk for developing panic disorder. Students who experience panic attacks frequently seek help from their physician or the emergency department before they present to a mental health provider, although these days more students are educated about panic and may first come to a counseling center. Panic symptoms are nonspecific and can signal any anxiety disorder, a mood disorder, a substance use disorder, or, more rarely in the college-aged population, a physical health problem. Sometimes they're situational and self-limited, and educating the student about the nature of the symptoms can prevent the anticipatory anxiety about having more panic, preventing the progression to panic disorder.

Panic also often accompanies various phobias, such as fear of flying. Students who present with the latter sometimes have quite constrained college experiences because of their fears: they may drive cross-country to school rather than fly, and avoid semester- or summer-abroad experiences or limit their postgraduate plans based on avoiding flight. Students who develop agoraphobia while on campus can suffer significant academic consequences, skipping class and being perceived as unmotivated.

The college years are considered a high-risk time for exposure to traumatic experiences as well. In surveys, most college students report having experienced at least one traumatic event when the definition of trauma includes death or life-threatening illness of a loved one or accidents. Most of these students, however, don't develop the difficult and sometimes debilitating symptoms of post-traumatic stress disorder (PTSD). Interestingly, there's a discrepancy between the types of trauma that students consider "worst" and the traumas that seem to cause the most symptoms. Sexual assault caused the greatest incidence of PTSD in one large study of college students, yet of the students who'd experienced it, only slightly more than a third rated it as their "worst ever" trauma.[14] Women and racial minority students reported more lifetime traumatic events than male and white students, highlighting the need to remain sensitive to differential risk among different students.

Since the number of international students on campus has dramatically increased, and since some of these students hail from regions of the world with significant violence or war, we may also see increases in PTSD among this student subgroup, though systematic research is lacking. And as more American-born students travel to regions of the world that are in conflict, or return to campus after serving in the Gulf wars, we may see increases in students suffering combat-related PTSD. Academic programs that immerse undergraduate students in different cultures sometimes inadvertently also expose them to experiences of vicarious traumatization, without adequate emotional preparation in advance or opportunities for debriefing once they return to campus. For example, one young student who returned from an academic experience where she interviewed women who'd survived an ethnic cleansing experience had significant psychological symptoms long after her return to campus, even though she didn't experience or directly witness the traumatic events.

Treatment Considerations

The good news for both Mike and Louise in the vignettes above is that there are several evidence-based treatment approaches for anxiety disorders, and early intervention often changes the entire course of a student's progression through school. For all students, the opportunity to discuss their fears and learn healthier ways of responding to them is invaluable. Of course, specific treatment will depend on the specific nature and severity of the problem. Because there is so much diagnostic overlap between the anxiety disorders, I worry less about a specific diagnostic code and instead try to understand the nature and patterns of the anxiety.

If a student's anxiety seems short lived and mostly situational, then simple relaxation techniques, breathing exercises, and reassurance may be all that's needed. Education about the nature of anxiety and how avoidance reinforces it, while action and exposure can extinguish it also goes a long way with intelligent, self-motivated students. Some of these interventions can be delivered in a group format. At Duke we regularly offer brief (one- to three-session) workshops on "worrying well" and stress management. We also offer regular mindfulness meditation groups, and although these are not specifically targeted to anxiety, they often significantly reduce worry. Advertising these to the entire campus community, rather than reserving these groups only for clinicians' referrals, allows a broader range of students to participate and to benefit.

Even in students dealing with situational or short-lived anxiety, if sleep impairment is present, then we address it directly. Sometimes a focus on sleep hygiene will be sufficient (with written instructions to the student), but sometimes, a short course of either a hypnotic agent or a low-dose benzodiazepine is invaluable in breaking a cycle of worry and insomnia. Because college students with anxiety frequently turn to alcohol or drugs as coping mechanisms, any comorbid substance use must be addressed through a combination of education and motivational interviewing.

A student like Mike or Louise likely needs a more intensive treatment approach. CBT is effective for all the anxiety disorders. Specific manualized treatments for each disorder can be helpful, as can group treatment approaches. Although the evidence is strongest for CBT groups, for college students, attending to group dynamics may be equally effective. One small study comparing a CBT group for social anxiety to a control group psychotherapy approach based on Yalom and Leszcz found that the control group did just as well on all measures of improvement in social anxiety and actually had less attrition.[15] The control group used more nonspecific group interventions, such as encouraging participants to support each other, and provide feedback on how they perceived each other, and take responsibility for group participation and homework assignments. My own clinical experience resonates with this finding: many socially anxious students have benefitted from general group therapy experiences over the years, including interpersonal groups, grad groups, dissertation support groups, and others, especially when CBT groups specifically targeting anxiety or social anxiety were not available. Since social interactions with peers are such an important developmental task for emerging adults, it makes sense that the exposure to the nonspecific components of group processes, and the ability to receive feedback in the moment, are invaluable to students—once they are finally persuaded to go!

For students with PTSD, those treatments that include some element of an exposure-based CBT are likely to be most helpful, based on recommendations of a 2007 Institute of Medicine review of evidence-based therapies. These exposure-based CBTs include cognitive reprocessing therapy and eye-movement desensitization and reprocessing (EMDR).[16]

Many psychotropic medications are helpful in treating anxiety (table 14.1). Some therapists suggest that psychotherapy should be the first-line treatment, since it's been proven to be effective and safe and since its benefits may last longer after the completion of treatment than those of medications. I believe that the decision regarding therapy or medicine (or both) should be guided by the student's level of distress and impairment, personal and family mental health history, and student preference. A concern is that if a medication is helpful, the student may then have to take that medication indefinitely to maintain wellness. Students themselves, especially anxious students, also worry a lot about dependence on medicine and possible side effects. Anxious students tend to be more worried about taking any medicine and are so attuned to every side effect that it can be hard to simply have a medication trial of adequate dose and duration. Their concerns are all valid and should be addressed respectfully and comprehensively.

When a student prefers to start with psychotherapy and has access to it, that

Table 14.1   Pharmacological treatment of anxiety disorders

Anxiety disorder	First-line treatment	Alternatives	Adjuvant
Generalized anxiety disorder	SSRIs venlafaxine ER	buspirone	clonazepam lorazepam
Social anxiety disorder	SSRIs (esp. sertraline, escitalopram, fluvoxamine)	venlafaxine ER fluoxetine	clonazepam alprazolam beta-blockers for performance anxiety
PTSD	SSRIs SNRIs	phenelzine	risperidone prazosin
OCD	SSRIs, clomip-ramine	venlafaxine ER	atypical antipsychotics?*
Panic disorder	SSRIs SNRIs (venla-faxine ER, duloxetine)	tricyclics	alprazolam clonazepam lorazepam (consider standing dose at first)

Source: Adapted from Guideline Watch. (2013, March). *APA practice guidelines for the treatment of patients with obsessive-compulsive disorder;* Guideline Watch. (2009, March). *Practice guideline for the treatment of patients with acute stress disorder and posttraumatic stress disorder* and *Practice guideline for the treatment of patients with panic disorder* (2nd ed.); and Swinson, R. P., Antony, M. M., & Bleau, P. B., et al. (2006). "Clinical Practice Guidelines: Management of Anxiety Disorders." *Canadian Journal of Psychiatry, 51* (suppl. 2): 1–92.

*The evidence is mixed for atypical antipsychotic treatment of OCD.

is a wonderful first option. Some students have so much anxiety, however, that they can't meaningfully participate in the therapy process. At other times a student lacks sufficient time before an important anxiety-triggering event, such as final exams, to allow therapy to adequately take effect. In these cases I try to ease the student's fears by providing a lot of information about how and why medicines can help, along with my strong professional recommendation (rather than simply providing information on all options and asking the student to make the decision). I always remind them that the choice to take the medicine is entirely theirs, and that they can also choose to stop it at any point.

When treating an anxious student with any medicine, I start low and go slow: low initial dose and slow upward titration to minimize possible side effects. The SSRIs have all shown efficacy in treating GAD, social anxiety disorder, panic disorder, OCD, and PTSD. In general, higher doses usually work better for OCD-spectrum disorders and for PTSD than the doses that seem effective for depression, and it often takes longer to reach the therapeutic effect (for social anxiety disorder and OCD, as long as 8 to 12 weeks). When students have depression comorbid with obsessional symptoms, the depression sometimes improves before the anxiety. Conversely, some very anxious depressed students feel more relaxed starting medicine before they notice mood improvement. Some believe that less severe symptoms improve first.

Short-term use of low-dose, high-potency benzodiazepines can also help students without a history of alcohol or substance abuse, though in PTSD, benzodiazepines can sometimes worsen symptoms. I explain to students the conditioning power of anxiety, and how the fear of loss of control over fear can become a self-fulfilling prophecy. For many students, it's then sufficient to carry around their benzodiazepine and know they can take it if overwhelmed; we discuss this, and often they then find that they don't need to take it.

Although beta blockers were not found to be particularly effective in generalized social anxiety disorder, they can be extremely helpful in cases of disabling performance anxiety. Their use allows students to participate more easily in exposure to feared situations, which ultimately reduces the fear.

Students with a history of significant trauma usually do best in a setting that doesn't impose the kinds of length-of-treatment limits that most college counseling centers must impose. However, sometimes barriers to other care leave the counseling center as the student's only treatment option. In those instances, brief treatment may serve as a bridge to more comprehensive treatment, or medication can provide symptom stabilization.

CHAPTER 15

Depression and Other Mood Problems

Many of the students described in previous vignettes listed depressive symptoms along with their other concerns, because mood complaints are common on campus. Determining whether a student has a mood disorder, or mood lability linked to another psychiatric diagnosis, or simply variability in mood due to normal life stressors can be challenging. Students sometimes complain directly of depression, or sad or low mood, or of a history of depression that keeps them vigilant to changes in their level of functioning. But it's just as common for them to present a relationship difficulty, or homesickness, or physical complaints, and then reveal mood symptoms later or subtly during the evaluation. Occasionally, depressed students come to our attention via the concern of a faculty member or a friend.

Diagnosing Depression

Jamal is emergently referred to the counseling center by his academic dean after several of his professors expressed concerns over his class absences. Fifteen minutes late to the appointment, this 20-year-old African American sophomore smells of cigarette smoke and has disheveled hair. He admits that he's been sleeping much of the day because he's had difficulty sleeping at night. His speech is quiet and sparse, his eye contact intermittent, and he reports skipping classes because he's been doing poorly and is too embarrassed to face his professors. In fact, he's not talking much to anyone, mostly keeping to himself in his room. He skips meals and has lost about 10 pounds. He'd returned this semester from a medical leave of absence for appendicitis but notes a similar pattern prior to the leave: "I'd stopped going to classes then too, and would've flunked out probably but had to have surgery right before finals so I got to go on medical leave instead." He wonders if he's just not smart enough for college and feels helpless, hopeless, and worthless. He sometimes bangs his head against the wall in frustration with himself, notes he's recently taken up smoking but denies other self-harm thoughts or actions. He admits that if a car were to hit him, however, "it wouldn't be the end of the world."

Depression may occur more frequently among college students than among the general U.S. population. One study found that one in four students was depressed during the previous year, and that men and women were about equally affected (unlike in the general population).[1] College students reportedly sought help for depression twice as often in 2000 as students had 13 years previously.[2] Students cite academic difficulties as one of the most common precipitants of depressive symptoms, but it's hard to know which came first, since depression clearly causes severe impairment in academic performance. In fact, about 92% of students diagnosed with depression or dysthymia at a large midwestern university experienced academic impairment, defined as missed academic time from class, decreased academic productivity, and significant interpersonal problems at school.[3] This is higher than the work impairment usually reported for adults with depression.

Students who begin to do poorly academically often reason that they feel down and demoralized because of their poor performance, and certainly that's possible. But students who, like Jamal, show a longer course of deteriorating mood and function, and who also have neurovegetative symptoms, likely are suffering from a treatable mood disorder. Treating the depression won't necessarily help them salvage their academic semester, but not treating it will certainly lead to failure.

African American college students are at increased risk of depression, yet they also typically tend to underutilize campus counseling and other mental health services due to various cultural factors.[4] Cultural barriers may also deter students from other countries and from certain religious and ethnic backgrounds from viewing mood problems as a mental health issue. It's therefore especially important to design effective outreach programs and to educate faculty and other campus staff who come in regular contact with students to ensure that students don't fall through the cracks.

Jamal's history presents several areas of concern that require further investigation. First, he's suffered similar symptoms in the past without addressing them, raising the possibility of a more chronic depression, such as dysthymia, or a recurrent major depression. Second, his self-critical stance, social isolation, hopelessness, and passive suicidal thoughts put him at risk for self-harm, and a careful risk assessment is critical. African American students have lower suicide rates than white students, but some scholars suggest these data are outdated, since the proportion of African Americans in college has grown since the information was collected in the late 1990s; in the intervening years, some studies have shown escalating rates of suicidal behavior among African American male adolescents.[5] Also, some report a higher rate of suicide among students who have dropped out of college, suggesting that someone like Jamal, who is at risk of failing out, may be at an especially critical risk juncture. This juncture is also an invaluable opportunity for receiving treatment.

Jamal becomes more forthcoming once the interviewer empathizes with how uncomfortable it might be for him to talk about personal problems with a stranger at an adviser's request. The psychiatrist also asks about the attitudes toward mental health treatment in the student's family and town. Jamal grew up in a largely African American southern community and admits that college was a culture shock. In some of his classes he is the only nonwhite student, leading him to feel like he reflects poorly on his race when he "messes up." He has no significant past psychiatric history, but began to feel somewhat apathetic his freshman year after feeling overwhelmed with schoolwork. He began to smoke marijuana, and then tobacco as he tried to fit in with various social groups. He noticed worsening concentration and sleep problems, began to skip classes, and then suffered the appendicitis that led to his leave. While home recovering from his appendectomy he divulged to no one how poorly he'd been doing, nor did he or anyone else suggest he might be depressed.

He worked at a restaurant over the summer and his sleep and appetite improved, but he admits, "I never felt back to my regular self," no longer feeling entirely at home with his old friends or with family, but also feeling disconnected and fearful about college. He is unaware of any family history of depression, but his father was alcoholic. His parents divorced when he was five and never attended college. He is estranged from his father and was raised by his mother and her parents, who are "very religious." In college he has felt more distant from his church and guilty about this as well.

There's a better appreciation these days of the difficulties faced by first-generation students as they navigate the transition to college. In evaluating these students, and especially when a student is also from an underrepresented racial or ethnic group on campus, one that has historically been exposed to racism, it's important to remain sensitive to the normal dysphoria or difficulties any student in that situation would face while still evaluating for the possibility of a psychiatric problem that would benefit from focused treatment. Severity and duration of symptoms and level of impairment can help make this distinction. When a student has already gone on a leave of absence for similar problems, clearly the level of impairment is high. Jamal concluded, as do many students who struggle academically, that he's not cut out for college, or for this particular college. These feelings come up even with students who are not first-generation college students or from minority groups; they come up with graduate and professional school students as well. But given the nature of university admissions, most students have clearly demonstrated that they have the capacity to do university work—something is likely interfering. By the time a student like Jamal comes to our attention, depressive symptoms and academic underperformance are so entangled that it's impossible to help the student answer questions of fit with his university right away. I usually recommend that we address the depression, then assess academic performance, and after that, make a decision regarding staying in school, or at a particular school.

The overlap between depression, anxiety disorders, and substance abuse is significant. Students frequently address their dysphoria through alcohol or marijuana, but alcohol and other drug abuse can also exacerbate or cause dysphoria, clouding the diagnostic picture. Jamal has several other risk factors associated with college student depression: poor grades, a sense of not belonging, cigarette smoking, and the use of illegal drugs.[6] Jamal's use of cannabis, if frequent enough and heavy enough, may have precipitated an amotivational syndrome that looks very much like depression but would not respond to treatment while he continues to use. Depressed or suicidal college students are at greater risk of nonmedical prescription drug use as well, including painkillers, antidepressants, and stimulants.[7] Female students in particular self-medicate inappropriately with painkillers.

As we evaluate students with depressive symptoms, it's also helpful to ask about seasonal variability, which could signal a seasonal affective disorder. DSM-5 includes the specifier "with seasonal pattern" for depressive episodes that clearly occur mostly at a specific time of year and notes that these are often characterized by hypersomnia, energy, overeating and weight gain, and craving for carbohydrates. For women, depression or irritability associated with the luteal phase of the menstrual cycle, about seven to ten days before the onset of menses, suggests premenstrual dysphoric disorder.

Bipolar Spectrum?

When a diagnosis of depression seems likely, the next step is to consider whether it is a unipolar or bipolar variant. Bipolar disorders have been separated from depressive disorders in the DSM-5, to reflect their place "as a bridge" between psychotic disorders and depressive disorders in terms of symptoms and genetics. Students rarely present in a manic or hypomanic state, although this can happen. Mania, with its pressured speech, inappropriate and labile affect, and frequent delusional content, is fairly easy to diagnose during a clinical assessment. More difficult is to identify mania and especially hypomania by history in college students. The college lifestyle is so erratic that reports of sleep disruption or bouts of increased energy are the norm.

Most college students seen for mental health evaluation also endorse racing thoughts or times of increased impulsivity if asked. In my experience, students who describe racing thoughts are more commonly experiencing anxiety rather than mania or hypomania. Asking for specific examples can help because these can be evaluated by comparison to the norms within their university community. It's important to know too whether mood swings are precipitated by substance use, especially stimulants, cocaine, marijuana, or alcohol. Collateral information from roommates, friends, or family is also helpful, if the student gives permission. Family history is useful but not definitive, especially if it is negative. Because bipolar disorder is underdiagnosed in general, a family history of alcoholism, for example, may mask an undiagnosed bipolar (or depressive) spectrum illness in the family member.

Students often describe mood swings or sometimes even say, "I wonder if I'm manic-depressive because my mood changes so rapidly." These types of comments, when clarified, often don't describe states of true euphoria or depression; they usually reflect developmentally normal mood reactivity to interpersonal or academic situations, or the mood instability that sometimes accompanies a personality disorder. The intensity, duration, and consequences of the mood states are all critical diagnostic clues. Some mental health professionals suggest that the triad of psychotic symptoms, hypersomnia, and diurnal mood variation, especially when accompanied by shorter and more frequent depressive episodes, points to a bipolar rather than unipolar depression.[8]

Screening scales such as the Mood Disorders Questionnaire or the Young Mania Rating Scale can help identify students at risk for bipolar disorder, but they cannot make a definitive diagnosis. They also can help track a student's response to treatment.

Other Diagnostic Considerations in Students

Although both major depressive disorder and bipolar disorder have a mean age of onset right during the college years, many students with depressive symptoms, and even with some hypomanic symptoms, will likely not go on to have chronic major psychiatric illnesses; the numbers of students presenting with these complaints are in excess of the prevalence rates of these disorders in the general population. So an ongoing challenge is to identify and treat those students whose illness might become severe, while not overtreating the rest. For example, one longitudinal study of college students who had scored high on the Hypomanic Personality Scale (HYP) found that more of these people had bipolar disorder or depression compared with a control group when interviewed (by structured interview) 13 years later. Of the HYP group, 25% had diagnoses of bipolar disorder at follow-up, compared with none of the control group, and 28% experienced a unipolar depressive disorder, compared with 19% in the control group.[9] So, clearly the high scorers in college were at significantly increased risk, but about half of them did not progress to a full-blown psychiatric disorder. This suggests that it's important to treat aggressively when the diagnosis is clear, but perhaps to be cautious when it's less clear, since the medications for depression and especially for bipolar disorder carry their own health risks.

Another challenge to accurately diagnosing depression in college students may reflect the brain maturation that is now known to continue into the early to mid-twenties. The frontal lobes, and the frontolimbic system, have been implicated in depression, and these are areas that reach full maturity later.[10] Adolescents process emotions differently than adults do, with increasing control by the frontal lobes as they mature.[11] So the emotional volatility seen in some students may represent a lag in neurobiological maturation, which will resolve with time. In those cases, we wouldn't want to start a medication that the student would have to continue indefinitely.

The college years are a time of tremendous situational change. Students' lives are changing not only on campus, semester to semester, but sometimes also at home. Some students who present with mood symptoms may be experiencing an adjustment disorder. Others are experiencing grief or bereavement. Some may be suffering from a personality disorder, but again, because so much change characterizes this group, what looks like a personality disorder in a college freshman may have changed or disappeared by senior year as the student matures. As always, establishing a strong therapeutic alliance while doing a comprehensive assessment helps facilitate collaborative treatment planning.

Treatment Approaches for Mood Symptoms in Students

It's important to get the best possible diagnostic clarity at the time of initial evaluation, including target symptoms and goals for treatment, while keeping in mind that there's considerable diagnostic overlap and symptom fluidity in this population. This means an important component of treatment is continued reassessment, and recognition that the full diagnostic picture may not be available at intake or may change as the student progresses through developmental stages.

Many college counseling centers work in a brief therapy model, with limits on the number of sessions available to students. About two-thirds of counseling centers across the country have access to on-campus psychiatric consultation,[12] leaving a third with no access to immediate psychiatric care, and in smaller communities, perhaps also limited access to psychiatric referral. Even in those instances, however, it's important to at least educate students about the full range of treatment options that exists for depression.

There's still what I consider an artificial distinction between "biological" treatments for mood disorders and "psychological" treatments. In fact, we know that the brain is continually modified by experience, and that psychotherapy is thus also a "biological" treatment. And taking a medication likewise has meaning and psychological consequences for most people. Therefore, in all psychiatric practice but perhaps especially with bright, curious college students, a holistic approach to treatment is most helpful, to address the complexity of how mood disruption affects mind, body, and spirit. Some students are looking for a quick fix to a complex problem and want only medication. Others fear medication and have been convinced that it never helps. Taking time to address these concerns and to design a holistic treatment plan should be the goal with each student.

Psychotherapy

Many forms of depression, adjustment problems, homesickness, and grief respond well to various forms of psychotherapy. Cognitive behavioral, interpersonal, and psychodynamic therapies all work well for university students. However, there isn't yet a clear "evidence base" of best therapies in the college population. The pace of college, where particular problems arise more frequently at certain times of the academic year, and where students come and go, makes it difficult to replicate exactly some of the treatments that have shown efficacy in other clinical settings. Across the country, students come for an average of five to six sessions of counseling, regardless of whether their center imposes session limits. Some studies suggest that the experience of the therapist, and other nonspecific variables such as the ability to form a therapeutic alliance, better predict good outcomes than does the theoretical orientation of the therapist.[13]

It's important to address issues that have particular relevance to the lives of students, including academic progress, relationship issues, and career choice. Depression and career indecision appear to be linked in college students, and similarly, positive affect seems to enhance a sense of self-efficacy.[14] When a student is performing poorly, as Jamal is in the vignette above, it's vital to spend some time problem solving with him regarding his academic situation. Students can be directed back to their deans or advisers to discuss their options, but depressed students often find it hard to take that step. A practical, problem-solving approach can sometimes be the best intervention. If a student is paralyzed by his depression, we might call the dean together from my office. At other times we brainstorm about options, including taking incompletes, withdrawals from one or two classes, or a medical leave from the university. Even if the student has already discussed these options with a dean or professor, viewing the possibilities through a therapeutic lens might give him a different perspective.

Pharmacotherapy

The SSRIs and the SNRIs are all about equally effective in treating major depressive episodes and can all be used as first-line medications in college students. Choice of a specific medicine thus depends on the student's history, family history of either good response to or problems with a particular medication, and side effect profiles. In my experience, college students especially want to avoid medicine that will make them sleepy or cause weight gain. Most also want to avoid sexual side effects, but the occasional young man with premature ejaculation finds this side effect helpful. Students are usually concerned about cost and prefer the least expensive generic medicines.

Although depressed students frequently use alcohol or illicit substances to cope, they are also often hesitant to take medication for their depression. It's not uncommon to spend multiple sessions with students before they decide to try medication. These times provide an opportunity to inject psychotherapy into the treatment, especially if the student has initially been reluctant about that option as well.

It's important to understand their concerns about taking medicine. Often they've read or heard something that is inaccurate. Some are afraid medicine will "change their personality." Some are afraid it will dull their intellect or sap their creativity. Some don't want to stop drinking. Some fear needing a "crutch," or worry they will have to take it forever. Providing psychoeducation, including, if possible, written materials, is critical. Students should understand the time lag between starting an antidepressant and experiencing its beneficial effects, as well as the usual duration of treatment. For many college students, the six- to nine-month window of treatment, followed by a gradual taper, is sufficient. Students with dysthymia, previous episodes of depression, or comorbid anxiety often do need longer treatment, but I always stress that this is their choice. If the diagnosis is bipolar disorder, then ongoing medication can prevent worsening of the illness over time. We always discuss alternative treatment options, as well as important complements to medicine. We discuss the importance of environmental changes, such as exercising more, practicing good sleep hygiene, and increasing social connections. And of course, avoiding alcohol and other drugs is critical, but given the prevalence of these on campus, abstaining can be a challenge.

Some students have already tried an antidepressant and had either bad side effects or no improvement. It's critical to get details about these trials, as more and more psychiatric medications are being prescribed by nonpsychiatrists and by clinicians under such time pressure that the student might not have been adequately educated about dose, duration, or side effects. Often the failed trials were too short to conclude anything, or a medicine was started at too high a dose, causing side effects that led the student to conclude she could never tolerate the medicine. Sometimes the opposite occurs: a student is maintained on a subtherapeutic dose of an antidepressant. Increasing the dose to therapeutic range sometimes produces a robust response.

The antidepressants carry warnings about possibly inducing suicidal thinking, especially in young people up to age 24. This can frighten students, and we always address it. In my experience, it's much more common for a student who has been suffering from suicidal ideation to experience its resolution once the medication is working, but once or twice a student has complained of new or more intense suicidal thoughts after starting an antidepressant. It's important to monitor all students closely once they've started a medicine, and in general to see them back within two weeks after beginning a trial.

Antidepressants can precipitate mania in vulnerable individuals, so prescribing them for students who have a family history of bipolar disorder or some suggestion of hypomania in their own history entails risk that must be discussed. Students with a bipolar diagnosis need treatment with mood stabilizers. Students presenting with acute mania usually need hospitalization, but if there's sufficient support for outpatient stabilization—for example, when parents come to stay with the student or there's a similar level of support and supervision from other family members or staff—the student can be treated with divalproate, or with several of the newer atypical antipsychotic medications, which have shown efficacy in randomized controlled trials. Lithium, though an excellent mood stabilizer, often has side effects that are intolerable to college students, including cognitive dulling, polyuria, tremor, and weight gain. Several anticonvulsants are good maintenance treatment options, but particularly lamotrigine, which has shown efficacy as a maintenance treatment[15] that seems well tolerated by students and is somewhat better than lithium or placebo at preventing depressive relapse. Students with a bipolar disorder diagnosis also need therapy to address the many issues raised by the diagnosis, including the need to make lifestyle modifications that are particularly hard to make as a college student.

Whether to start with psychotherapy, pharmacotherapy, or a combination of both depends on the severity and duration of symptoms, diagnosis, life disruption or impairment, patient history or past treatment response, and student preference. If the student has bipolar disorder, type I, or a severe depression with psychotic symptoms, then medication should be the first-line treatment.

Other Considerations

Students with depression, dysthymia, or bipolar disorder may need help beyond therapy, medication, and lifestyle modification. Some universities now have deans who serve case worker functions, and involving these individuals in a student's care (with the student's permission) allows a comprehensive response to the student's needs. These deans can arrange for academic relief, accommodations where appropriate, and on-campus support to reduce risk. They can also follow students longitudinally. Often students with chronic or severe problems are referred off campus for ongoing treatment. Case managers can help ensure that the referral "sticks"; otherwise, there is significant risk that the student won't follow through with recommended treatment and will deteriorate. Most university counseling centers work with a network of off-campus clinicians who have extensive experience working with college students and are well-versed in coordinating with campus resources. Our center actually developed the position of a "referral coordinator" to help students find and maintain the treatment relationships they need and to help them navigate the often bewildering morass of insurance issues that can emerge.

Some, such as former University of Virginia's counseling center director Russ Federman, argue that students with bipolar disorder are best cared for within the counseling center. Federman suggests that the ideal treatment setting is a system of care that integrates brief psychotherapy with pharmacotherapy, addresses the normal developmental denial that many bipolar students experience, and provides support groups.[16] He also notes that the university community can more easily monitor and respond to the rapid changes in mood that can occur with bipolar disorder. I agree that having this integrated system of care is the ideal treatment for many students with mood disorders. Unfortunately, many schools lack the resources, and in their absence, it's best to seek appropriate referrals for ongoing care where it exists.

Whether to medicate students with depression before they've committed to sobriety can seem like a dilemma. Certainly heavy alcohol or cannabis use can cause a substance-induced mood disorder, distinct from major depression, which would likely clear with abstinence. Prescribed stimulants, if abused, and cocaine can precipitate manic-like states. Most students will agree to at least a trial period of abstinence to clarify their diagnosis, but it's often hard to convince them to spend the 30-day substance-free period that the literature recommends to distinguish substance-induced from independent mood disorders.

Research increasingly highlights the high rate of independent depression even among people with substance dependence. In university populations, it's more the exception to find a student with depression who abstains from alcohol. More likely, a student has an independent mood disorder and also uses substances in the way that many of her peers do. The decision about prescribing medicine should then involve careful weighing of risks versus benefits. When alcohol or substance abuse is comorbid with depression, both problems are more severe and often more entrenched. Recent evidence questions the wisdom of withholding medication while people are still using, since medication improves both the depressive symptoms and the substance use.[17] Careful, judicious treatment of mood symptoms even in the context of continuing substance use can help improve mood symptoms enough that the student can make better use of therapy and reduce reliance on alcohol and drugs. Of course, a student who meets criteria for moderate to severe alcohol or substance use disorders likely needs a higher level of care than outpatient treatment, with a specialized dual diagnosis focus.

For a student like Jamal, ideal treatment would involve practical problem solving at the outset—help with academic relief, deciding whether to take medical leave, and considering whether tutoring or other academic assistance might help—and then a combination of antidepressant medication and psychotherapy. I'd regularly assess and address his marijuana and tobacco use and use motivational interviewing techniques to help him move toward relinquishing these. If Jamal chose to take medical leave, I'd work to identify a psychiatrist in his hometown and make some follow-up phone calls to encourage him to follow through with treatment. If he remained on campus, I'd identify groups he might join to diminish his sense of isolation, including any existing forums for first-generation college students, groups based on his religious affiliation (if he continues to value that part of his identity) or his background, and groups based on academic or extracurricular interests.

The majority of students with depression, dysthymia, or other mood complaints improve with outpatient treatment. Many students with bipolar disorder, if engaged in regular treatment, also do quite well, though mania or psychotic symptoms may require hospitalization to stabilize.

CHAPTER 16

Psychotic Symptoms

Adalet is a 23-year-old Turkish international graduate student in her first year of a comparative literature program. She comes in at the urging of her roommate, an Argentinian international student with whom she was randomly paired. The roommate accompanies Adalet to the session and states, "I think she's suffering from a broken heart and needs some therapy." Adalet has fallen in love with Joe, an American student in her program, but according to the roommate, "He doesn't seem to know that she exists." Lately Adalet has been eating less, not showering, and not going to classes. She listens quietly to her roommate's concerns and then asks the roommate to leave. She is casually dressed, but her hair is greasy and disheveled. Her voice is soft and speech is sparse and initially guarded. When asked to describe Joe, she becomes animated, and her affect becomes joyous. She is convinced he loves her and that she will marry him, and she blames herself for inadvertently missing his previous cues that he was interested. For example, she noticed that he changed his Facebook status to indicate where he was going last Friday night, and in retrospect she knows this was a direct invitation to her alone to join him, but she did not. This is how she explains his avoidance of her now in class and his lack of response to her phone calls or texts. She describes several other ideas of reference. She denies depressive symptoms but admits that she has not been sleeping well and is not concentrating in class. However, she expects she will do well in her classes because she can "sense" more information than her peers and sees connections they miss. She shares a literary interpretation that is illogical and demonstrates looseness of associations; she sadly adds that her professor isn't smart enough to see the brilliance of her work. She has no past psychiatric history, denies any substance use, and is unaware of psychiatric problems in her family, who live in Turkey.

Elliot, an 18-year old Caucasian freshman, is brought in urgently by his mother, who came to campus after her son sounded "completely off" in a phone call, "talking nonsense." She then spoke with one of his fraternity brothers, who said they'd noticed Elliot seemed more anxious lately, saying "weird stuff." Elliot admits he'd been smoking marijuana a lot recently and had begun to feel anxious and paranoid after intoxication the previous week. However, he denies any use since then. Urine drug screen is positive only for THC. There is no past psychiatric history. He has some awareness that others don't understand what he's been saying, and states, "It may be because people think I have a chip in my head. I do have a photographic memory, you know." He is flushed and appears anxious on exam, easily becoming argumentative, especially with his mother. His mother asks whether this is caused by marijuana and whether her son needs to be taken to rehab.

Most students experiencing psychotic symptoms—hallucinations, delusions, paranoia, or grossly disorganized thinking—come to psychiatric attention when others are concerned. Sometimes additional symptoms or flagging school performance bring them in. They may be aware that something is wrong but often lack the insight to consider the psychotic symptoms themselves to be a medical or psychiatric problem. Some may fear that if they reveal their symptoms, they will be labeled crazy. Because major psychotic illnesses, such as schizophrenia, are so disruptive and cognitively disabling, it's rare for students to arrive at college or graduate school with a poorly controlled psychotic disorder. It's also rare for the presence of psychotic symptoms to actually signal the start of a major psychotic disorder in this population, but when they do, quick diagnosis and treatment are essential.

Prevalence rates of psychotic disorders specifically in college students are hard to come by. The 2012 Healthy Minds Study of more than 20,000 students at 29 institutions found a self-reported incidence of about 0.1% for schizophrenia and about 0.2% for other psychotic disorders.[1] In 2011–2012 outcome data at the counseling center at Duke University, clinicians reported a "psychotic episode" diagnosis in 6 of 1607 students seen, or less than 0.4%. However, psychotic *symptoms* among emerging adults are a different story. The young seem prone to occasional unusual experiences. In community samples of young adolescents, 21% report having heard voices or sounds, yet the majority don't have psychotic illnesses.[2] Those adolescents do, however, have higher rates of other emotional difficulties. Furthermore, most appear to outgrow psychotic symptoms, so their occurrence later in adolescence may be more ominous— though again, more commonly linked to nonpsychotic illnesses. In a large birth-cohort sample of New Zealand emerging adults ages 18 to 23, those with major depressive disorder or an anxiety disorder had a fivefold greater incidence of psychotic symptoms compared to those without, even when numbers were adjusted for alcohol or other substance use.[3]

Among college students, isolated psychotic symptoms might be quite common. Differentiating between clinically significant and more benign ones may depend on frequency of symptoms and whether they cause distress. One study examined the use of a self-report psychotic symptoms questionnaire (the Prodromal Questionnaire) in a nonclinical sample of over 1,000 undergraduates enrolled in psychology classes.[4] When the researchers used a previously validated cut-off of eight positive symptoms to suggest a need for further clinical evaluation, 43% of the sample screened positive. If in addition these symptoms had to be frequent, as in weekly, the positive percentage dropped to 8%, and it dropped even further, to 2%, when including the requirement that symptoms be "distressing." Most of these students had not sought help for their symptoms, though a greater number in this last category had. This study suggests that some psychotic symptoms are a common experience for nearly half of undergrads at one time or another, and that they rarely cause these students to seek help. Population screening might nevertheless help identify those students for whom these symptoms are evolving into serious concerns—and allow access to earlier treatment.

Diagnostic Considerations

The challenge in working with students is neither to overreact, inappropriately treating someone whose psychotic symptoms are relatively harmless, nor to miss those who are actually in the midst of a "first break" of psychosis. It's increasingly clear that early detection and treatment of schizophrenia leads to

Table 16.1   Attenuated psychosis syndrome

A. At least one of the following symptoms are present in attenuated form, with relatively intact reality testing, and is of sufficient severity or frequency to warrant clinical attention:
1. Delusions
2. Hallucinations
3. Disorganized speech
B. Symptom(s) must have been present at least once per week for the past month.
C. Symptom(s) must have begun or worsened in the past year.
D. Symptom(s) is sufficiently distressing and disabling to the individual to warrant clinical attention.
E. Symptom(s) is not better explained by another mental disorder, including a depressive or bipolar disorder with psychotic features, and is not attributable to the physiological effects of a substance or another medical condition.
F. Criteria for any psychotic disorder have never been met.

Source: American Psychiatric Association. (2013). *Diagnostic and statistical manual of mental disorders,* 5th ed. (DSM-5). Washington, D.C.: American Psychiatric Association.
    Note: This syndrome is recommended for further study in section 3 of the DSM-5.

better outcomes: fewer negative symptoms, less depression and cognitive impairment, and even higher rates of full recovery.[5] For these reasons, researchers working on DSM-5 considered including a diagnostic category for "psychosis risk syndrome," but this was understandably controversial. Broadening a diagnosis to include risk might have led to unnecessary treatment of too many people, as well as incorrectly labeling people with a diagnosis that unfortunately still carries stigma. Instead, the category of "attenuated psychosis syndrome" is included in the "Conditions for Further Study" section of DSM-5, recognizing the mix of symptoms we sometimes struggle to diagnose and suggesting a need for further research (see table 16.1).[6] Between 20% and 50% of patients who are evaluated as having attenuated psychosis syndrome at specialty prodrome clinics progress to a psychotic illness within a year, so students who meet these diagnostic criteria need close monitoring. The question of best treatment in those cases is not yet fully clear.

It's rare for psychotic symptoms in college students to signify schizophrenia. More commonly they herald the onset of a delusional disorder or are part of a mood disorder, such as bipolar or unipolar depression; an anxiety disorder, such as PTSD; or another psychiatric problem. Also rare in healthy young adults, but not impossible, is that psychosis is part of a medical condition. Among college students, substance use is a common trigger. Frequent cannabis users are at doubled risk for schizophrenia and increased risk for psychotic symptoms in general.[7] Presentations like Elliot's are a common way for psychotic symptoms to come to clinical attention.

Of course, it's hard to say definitively whether a student like Elliot experienced psychotic symptoms because of the marijuana, or whether he started to use drugs in response to the emergence of paranoia or anxiety. More and more, neurobiological data suggest that drugs trigger symptoms in genetically vulnerable individuals, with earlier exposure being more harmful. The endocannabinoid system in the brain is involved in regulating energy states, cognition, emotional responses, motor control, and motivated behavior, and it seems to be especially sensitive to disruptions earlier in life.[8] Case reports document examples of college students without previous psychiatric problems who experienced psychotic symptoms and ultimately bipolar disorder after cannabis use.[9] Unfortunately, simply detoxifying from the substance doesn't always result in remission of symptoms once they've been triggered. Treatment with antipsychotic medicine is often necessary.

Psychotic symptoms occur everywhere in the world, but their evaluation requires cultural astuteness. Some beliefs which seem delusional or bizarre to Western clinicians may be in keeping with a student's culture of origin. Occasionally a language barrier makes symptoms sound more ominous than they are, and a translator becomes an essential part of the work-up. When evaluating an international student for the possibility of psychosis, especially a student like Adalet, who presents with what appear to be delusions of an erotomanic subtype, it's important to ask about norms for her belief in her home country. What are her previous romantic experiences? What are the family's expectations? How firmly does Adalet believe that Joe, with whom she's had little contact, is in love with her and will marry her? Is she expressing a wish more than a belief? Is it possible that her symptoms are caused by sleep deprivation? Is any corroborating information available? Sometimes, if an adviser or a dean has gotten involved, many different people on campus are collecting reports of concerning behavior. The clinician can then discuss these with the student, in order to understand the student's thought processes and to assess insight and judgment. Conversely, with the student's permission, the clinician can help concerned people on campus understand which parts of a student's behavior are due to illness rather than willful misbehavior. In evaluating *any* student with psychotic symptoms, it's helpful to seek collateral information from peers, faculty, or family, especially regarding the student's functioning before psychotic symptoms started.

Adalet shares the text message she received from Joe a few days ago, before he stopped responding to her. It reads, "I can't have dinner or study together. Sorry." It's followed by a significant number of unanswered texts from her to him, but she dismisses these and emphasizes his expression of regret as a sign that he cares for her. She admits that two nights ago, she drove by his apartment building around midnight, saw him through his window, and when he didn't answer the door, she spent the night in the lobby, waiting for him to come out. In the morning he told her to go home and sleep, which "further proves that he cares for me." She denies any anger toward him or thoughts of wanting to hurt him or anyone else. She admits to slight concern over her declining academic performance, but adds, "That's a small price to pay for lifelong love, isn't it?"

Clearly Adalet is experiencing delusions and loss of insight. Her altered sleep and grandiosity suggest a possible mania diagnosis, although she denies a history of depression, and it would be unusual for bipolar disorder to present as mania. Her symptoms are causing behavior that is disturbing to her and to others in the university community. Although at this point the clinician evaluating Adalet has no knowledge of any formal complaints lodged by Joe, Adalet's pursuit of him may be considered stalking. In other, similar situations students have lodged complaints with university or local police. Risk assessment is critical. Although stalking *victims* on a university campus are much more frequently female and the perpetrators are more commonly male,[10] when the opposite is true, as in this vignette, it's even less likely that the victim will ask for help. Victims of stalking in college, compared to those in the general population, much less commonly report the crime, even though it often causes significant emotional consequences, including anxiety, depression, and obsessions.[11] Many campus stalkers have delays in social skills and lack abilities to navigate relationships; this may be the case for Adalet as well, but it cannot be fully evaluated while she is psychotic.

Sometimes, beginning treatment for psychotic symptoms with an antipsychotic medicine will help a student become more rational and facilitate better recall or articulation of other symptoms, especially mood problems. The distinction between a mood disorder with psychotic symptoms and a psychotic disorder is important, since it influences decisions about treatment options and treatment duration as well as prognosis.

Diagnostic evaluation in a student with new-onset psychotic symptoms should include blood tests: CBC, serum chemistries panel, liver function tests, thyroid-stimulating hormone, erythrocyte sedimentation rate, and a toxicology screen. A baseline EKG can be helpful if considering antipsychotic medication,[12] but it is not always necessary in healthy young adults with no family history of cardiac disease. Brain scans of otherwise healthy young adults, with no other indication of a neurological issue, are unlikely to benefit diagnosis or treatment, according to several reviews.[13] The scans may financially burden a student whose insurance does not fully cover the test and should probably be reserved for students who display neurological or other medical indication and perhaps for older students.

Treatment Considerations

If psychotic symptoms emerge incidentally during evaluation for another problem, and they don't seem frequent or distressing to the student, it is reasonable to focus first on the other issues while continuing to assess the psychotic symptoms. Because affective and anxiety disorders are much more common among college students, and the evidence suggests that psychotic symptoms are more often a part of these conditions than psychotic disorders, when anxiety or mood symptoms are present, we want to treat those along with the psychotic symptoms. For students like Adalet and Elliot, however, reducing psychotic symptoms must be the first goal of treatment.

Both Adalet and Elliot would likely benefit from antipsychotic medicine. But convincing students with limited insight to consider taking medicine that suggests they are "crazy" can often be extremely difficult, especially in the case of an international student who may have her own cultural biases against mental illness. There are no studies specifically on antipsychotic medicines in college students. However, studies on early intervention in adolescents and young adults at high risk for psychotic syndromes show that both pharmacotherapy and psychosocial treatments, such as CBT, significantly reduce the rate of subsequent psychosis compared with placebo.[14] Interestingly, some small prospective naturalistic studies suggest that treatment with antidepressants rather than antipsychotics in young people with prodromal symptoms actually leads to a lower rate of subsequent psychosis.[15] This is a very exciting possibility, since antidepressants generally have fewer adverse effects, are considered less stigmatizing, and are often cheaper. Adalet might not be a good candidate for an antidepressant given her lack of sleep, but in students with psychotic symptoms who resist taking an antipsychotic, antidepressants, especially combined with CBT that focuses on psychotic symptoms, might be a good treatment alternative.

I have gathered from my experience and from clinical discussions with colleagues that college students often respond to atypical antipsychotic medicine at lower doses than do older adults treated in other settings. Students sometimes improve quickly and dramatically, which may be in part due to the significant support networks they have, which most people with psychosis in the community lack. This allows for a more conservative treatment approach, and may thus make treatment more palatable. Starting low and titrating medicine slowly upward until symptoms either improve or resolve works well when peers, family, and faculty can also help monitor the student. Students are wary of side effects like sedation or cognitive slowing, and are usually averse to weight gain. Choosing a medicine that avoids these improves the likelihood that a student will adhere to treatment.

Difficulties arise when a student who is unwilling to take medication or participate in therapy is unable to attend class due to symptoms yet is not ill enough to justify involuntary treatment. International students present even greater complexity, since they usually lack family support, and any interruption in their schooling—for a medical leave, for example—often means they lose their student visa status and must go home. Some countries have limited psychiatric care options, and this raises ethical dilemmas about how to best care for such young people.

It can be invaluable to involve other campus professionals in collaborative treatment planning for psychotic students who have lost insight and are disruptive or in danger of deterioration without treatment. A dean or an adviser can help students think through options such as medical leave, withdrawal from a class, or modified workload. Sometimes a dean's assertion that a student can't continue in class without treatment motivates the student to accept clinical care. When psychotic symptoms lead to stalking, involvement of campus police and sometimes even local police becomes necessary. This requires balancing confidentiality with duty to protect; in such cases, consultation with colleagues is essential. Family involvement not only supports students while in treatment but also allows someone close to monitor for recurrence of symptoms once treatment has been discontinued. Most students with psychotic symptoms are in enough distress that they welcome and consent to their family's help. If psychosis persists or worsens, or if there's doubt about a student's adherence to treatment, hospitalization becomes unavoidable. College students often have incredible support and intellectual and emotional resources, however, so even hospitalized students can sometimes improve and return to school without having to take an extended leave of absence, though the option of medical leave must be considered whenever such serious problems arise.

Psychoeducation is important in working with this population, but it presents challenges. If we are still uncertain about diagnosis, not for lack of expertise but because these illnesses often take time to announce themselves, and in the beginning stages symptoms overlap, we don't want to unduly alarm a student by suggesting he has a major chronic psychotic illness that may interfere with his ability to complete school or pursue other goals. At the same time, it's important for students to understand the serious danger of psychotic symptoms, the possible illnesses into which these symptoms might evolve, and the risks of discontinuing treatment too early or, in some cases, at all. In the notorious Wendell Williamson case, Myron Liptzin, a college counseling center psychiatrist, treated Williamson, then a law student, for "delusional disorder" and recommended summer follow-up, including continued medications. Williamson did not comply with recommended treatment, and his psychosis recurred, leading to a shooting spree in which he killed two people. His diagnosis was later amended to schizophrenia, and he sued his psychiatrist and won, claiming the psychiatrist failed "to emphasize to the patient the severity of his disorder and its likely persistence, along with the need for lifelong use of medications."[16] The psychiatrist, the jury found, should have also made a more specific recommendation, naming another doctor for continued summer treatment. The decision was ultimately overturned, but it has led to increased caution in the way that follow-up treatment is recommended to students. Whether or not it has also led to increased use of antipsychotic medicine has not been systematically studied. But we should not allow fear of legal action to cloud our clinical judgment; instead use the principle "first, do no harm" in working with these complex questions in students.

All antipsychotic medicines have the potential for significant adverse effects, and the atypicals, which were supposed to be safer than the older "neuroleptics," have their own risk burden. Although they do appear to have lower risk of akathisia and tardive dyskinesia, they can cause metabolic syndrome, characterized by weight gain, lipid increases, and glucose intolerance,[17] which leads to poorer health. Whether these effects happen as frequently in young, otherwise healthy people isn't clear, but the possibility is concerning. Weight gain and prolactinemia is observed in some children and adolescents taking second-generation antipsychotics, even after controlling for developmentally normal weight gain and growth.[18] Not all the second-generation drugs carry the same level of risk: olanzapine appears to have the highest incidence, and aripiprazole and ziprasidone the lowest; risperidone is rated "mild." The newest medication, lurasidone, has a very low incidence of metabolic syndrome, but causes more akathisia and sedation than some of the others.[19] These are important considerations in choosing an antipsychotic for college students, although the medicines with the lower odds of weight gain and diabetes also cost significantly more than some of the other medicines, and cost is often an obstacle for students.

Because of the potential for metabolic side effects, several organizations, including the American Diabetes Association and the American Psychiatric Association, have issued guidelines for monitoring patients taking second-generation antipsychotic drugs and suggest that following the guidelines should be drug-driven, rather than dependent on diagnosis. Before beginning treatment with a second-generation antipsychotic, we should perform and record certain baseline assessments. These include reviewing personal and family history of coronary artery disease, diabetes, obesity, and hypertension; calculating BMI; and measuring waist circumference, fasting lipid panel, and fasting blood glucose. We can then monitor these periodically throughout treatment, although the available evidence is based on studies in adults, not college students (see table 16.2).

Table 16.2   Recommended monitoring in patients taking second-generation antipsychotic medications

Check at baseline	4 weeks	8 weeks	12 weeks	Quarterly	Annually	5 years
Personal/family history					X	
Weight & BMI	X	X	X	X		
Blood pressure			X		X	
Fasting lipid panel			X			X
Fasting blood glucose			X		X	
Waist circumference					X	

Source: Based on ADA and APA guidelines; American Diabetes Association. (2004). "Consensus Development Conference on Antipsychotic Drugs and Obesity and Diabetes." *Diabetes Care, 27,* 596–601.

These recommended steps are not routine in practice with college students. Perhaps because it is so rare to prescribe antipsychotics in this population, most of us don't have a system in place for monitoring. We may also fear that informing students of these risks will make them even less likely to take needed medication. But we need to protect our patients' health by monitoring and informing, especially as antipsychotic medicines are more frequently prescribed for nonpsychotic syndromes. There's some controversy over whose responsibility it is to monitor: the psychiatrist's or the primary care doctor's? It seems like good practice for psychiatrists to at the least recommend monitoring and appropriately refer. College students can be referred to the student health service, but then communication between the psychiatrist and student health center is critical. Significant changes in weight or other parameters should trigger consideration of nutritional counseling or changing medication.

In dealing with psychotic symptoms, college students anecdotally appear more resilient than young adults in other settings. This may be a reflection of the selection bias that allowed them to go on to higher education in the first place, or of their additional supports and resources. It would be extremely helpful to have more research in the future to help guide our treatment practices.

CHAPTER 17

Emergency Situations on Campus

An economics professor brings 19-year-old Marissa for an urgent counseling center evaluation, concerned because she broke into tears in his office after he'd called her in to discuss a failing grade. He reports that she'd been a strong student at the beginning of the semester but lately had been skipping class and not responding to e-mails, and now she'd failed an exam. Marissa told the professor that she'd been having personal problems and was in counseling. The record confirms that Marissa met twice with a psychology intern to discuss a flailing romantic relationship; there were no signs of high risk at that time. She no-showed to subsequent appointments and had not responded to the therapist's attempt to contact her.

During this evaluation, Marissa is initially reluctant to divulge much, saying, "This is so stupid. I'll be fine. I'm not crazy." She eventually admits that her boyfriend broke up with her two weeks ago, and she's felt unable to complete schoolwork since. She endorses multiple symptoms of depression but is ashamed, seeing everything as a sign of having been too dependent on her boyfriend. Her closest friend is on leave this semester, and she's felt isolated. This particularly bothers her since she already feels different from her peers due to the insulin-dependent diabetes she's had to manage since age 10. She admits, "Life is just too hard sometimes, and really doesn't seem worth it" and mumbles that she's thought about giving herself extra doses of insulin. She has been deterred by thoughts of how it would affect her mother. On the other hand, she says, "It would be easier on her to not have to figure out how to pay my tuition, now that I can't even get school right." Her parents went through a contentious divorce several years ago, and her father refuses to contribute to college expenses, "though financial aid is calculated based on both their incomes."

Emergency Assessment and Hospitalization

Psychiatrists assessing students in the midst of a crisis, whether in the counseling center or in other settings, must determine whether in addition to a high level of distress the student also is at risk of imminent harm, either to self or others. This is an imprecise science, made more difficult in the setting of work with emerging adults who may avoid fully disclosing symptoms for fear of being hospitalized, or simply because the achievement-oriented culture on many campuses actively discourages admitting or articulating vulnerability in general.

A variety of rating scales and assessment instruments have been studied in college populations, but none can in isolation predict risk. One of the more widely used scales, Beck's Scale for Suicidal Ideation (SSI), can be administered in about 10 minutes and has documented predictive validity for completed suicide.[1] When there's time, and if the student is willing to complete it, the SSI can be a helpful tool in risk assessment. The Counseling Center Assessment of Psychological Symptoms (CCAPS) scale, normed on college counseling center populations, also provides a helpful distress index and a hostility subscale in addition to symptom-related subscales;[2] norms are continually updated, and the instrument is available free of charge to university counseling centers (contact the Center for Collegiate Mental Health at Penn State). Many counseling centers use the CCAPS as an initial and a termination measure for all students seen there, and it can rapidly flag especially worrisome presentations.

Marissa presents several factors that elevate our concern for risk. She has insulin-dependent diabetes, considered one of the most psychologically challenging chronic medical conditions and one that doubles the risk of depression compared with the general population.[3] She has suicidal thoughts, articulates a plan, and has ready access to a potentially lethal means of self-harm (insulin overdose). She didn't adhere to treatment even before reaching crisis and did not seek help as she felt worse. She still lacks insight into the need for help. If she's suffering from untreated depression, her ability to adequately manage her diabetes may be compromised even in the absence of suicidal thoughts. Hospitalization would address both her mental and physical health needs.

When the psychiatrist suggests hospitalization to Marissa, she starts to weep and says, "It hasn't gotten to that point." The psychiatrist emphasizes the hospital as a place to stay safe, and Marissa retracts her previous self-harm statement, saying she won't "do anything stupid; I was just being a drama queen." She continues to make little eye contact. When asked if she's willing to engage in treatment outside the hospital she says, "Yeah, whatever."

Once a diagnosis of depression seems likely, a student who seems unengaged in assessment or treatment, who has expressed suicidal thoughts and a plan, and whose insight and judgment appear impaired needs a higher level of care than sporadic outpatient treatment, even if she changes her story once the discussion turns to hospitalization. Whether that higher level must include hospitalization is a decision that requires careful weighing of risks and benefits. If an alternative safety plan is available—for example, if a parent can come take custody of the student to ensure and monitor the student's physical safety and get the student to frequent outpatient appointments—then hospitalization can be averted in some cases. Sometimes a roommate, close friend, or residential staff member agrees to help supervise the student, but these arrangements are tricky. They place an undue burden on other students who may not know how to react in the event of clinical deterioration, or on non-clinically trained faculty. This doesn't eliminate risk and may simply delay inevitable hospitalization.

Other factors affect these decisions in work with students, such as the timing of the crisis within a semester. When a situation like the one above occurs close to the end of the semester, a safety plan that involves parental supervision and intensive outpatient work can get the student through the final week or weeks and prevent the loss of a semester's worth of work (and tuition!). Earlier in the semester, however, it may make more sense to take time off to focus entirely on treatment.

Absent other options, involuntary hospitalization may be necessary. Explaining this to the student occasionally convinces her to go voluntarily to the hospital, but not always. One study of more than 460,000 college students in Virginia found that in 2008–2009, the rate of hospitalization for psychiatric reasons was 6.82 per 10,000 students at public institutions, and 18.04 per 10,000 at private colleges; the rates of hospitalization based on college-initiated temporary custody or detention orders (involuntary hospitalization) was 4.97 (at public colleges) and 2.06 (at private ones).[4] A high proportion of hospitalized students, at least at public institutions, seems to have initially been unwilling to go. Hospitalization in general is rare, but it can be a life-saving intervention when illness severity and risk are high.

It's helpful for counseling centers to have protocols for both voluntary and involuntary student hospitalization. The JED Foundation has created the excellent *Framework for Developing Institutional Protocols for the Acutely Distressed or Suicidal College Student*, available at www.jedfoundation.org. This framework covers everything from who should respond to acutely distressed or suicidal students—and how—to issues around hospitalization, including how to transport students there. It also reviews who—and when—to notify and how to develop a post-crisis plan.

At Duke, our policy for voluntary hospitalization requires that trainees consult with their supervisors or the clinical director when considering hospitalization and specifies procedures for both office-hours and after-hours hospitalization. It recognizes that it's helpful to have two staff members working on hospitalization during office hours, so that one can handle logistics (e.g., phone calls to the emergency department, or to public safety) while the other attends to the student. Our involuntary hospitalization procedure lists some examples of situations and behaviors that might trigger the need for hospitalization and specifies that the staff member considering this must consult with a senior staff member or the clinical director, to ensure that all other less-restrictive options have been taken into account. It also recommends considering consultation with others outside the counseling center, such as deans or family members, and recognizes that involving family early, as appropriate, can help facilitate the student's longer-term care. Step-by-step procedures include which forms to fill out, what information is necessary, and the need to have campus police take commitment paperwork to the magistrate's office. These procedures will vary from school to school depending on state laws, university resources, and other factors, but thoughtfully crafting an appropriate response ahead of time allows a much more effective and efficient response in an emergency situation. Having a clear algorithm ensures an appropriate response even from staff members who may not remember all the steps because the situations in which they're needed are rare. Off-campus psychiatrists who routinely work with students should also periodically review their own familiarity with procedures for hospitalizing students.

Unfortunately, access to psychiatric care and hospitalization varies widely for college students. Some schools have a university hospital or affiliated medical center right on campus and have developed protocols that allow rapid student assessment and admission. Others are geographically far from inpatient services. Students may lack insurance coverage for psychiatric hospitalization, especially if they attend school outside their state of residence. All these factors affect the decision to hospitalize, but they should never trump risk assessment and actions that protect the student's—and others'—safety.

Depending on where the hospital is relative to the counseling center or private practitioner's office, transport can be a challenge when handling student emergencies. In some centers, counseling center staff members choose to walk students to the hospital or to accompany them on school or public transportation. This approach can have many therapeutic benefits, especially for younger undergraduate students who are far from home and for whom this represents a first encounter with the hospital. It also seems natural when the psychiatrist or therapist has a good therapeutic alliance with the student and wants to maintain and strengthen that alliance. Its main risk is that the student may change her mind and elope en route to the hospital, potentially then harming herself (or others). If accompanying the student means the psychiatrist has to cancel a full caseload of other students who need care, then this option may not be a good one.

There are no evidence-based guidelines on best practices for getting a student voluntarily to the hospital, but in my clinical experience most students don't want to go alone. Options include asking the student if a friend or family member is available to accompany him; identifying residential life staff who can do this; or, when a student is initially brought in by a faculty member, exploring whether that person feels comfortable taking the student to the hospital. Some students and faculty develop close relationships, and the support can be therapeutic. If there's any concern about safety, though, public safety officers should accompany the student. Policies on this vary across universities. Some officers will not transport students for psychiatric evaluation without involuntary commitment paperwork, which legally places the student in their custody. If the evaluating clinician is off campus, most campus police defer to the city police, and then response varies according to state laws. If a student has already hurt himself in some way, such as nonsuperficial cutting or taking an overdose, calling 911 for an ambulance immediately is the best course. Whenever we send a student emergently to the hospital, it's critical to communicate to the receiving clinician the clinical details that led us to recommend hospitalization.

A student who needs but refuses hospitalization presents challenges. On campus, public safety officers can wait with the student while we complete commitment paperwork. Some officers may insist that all paperwork be completed before they take the student into custody. We must do everything we can to ease the student's fears about hospitalization, especially when she's highly distressed or psychotic. It's very upsetting to a student when police officers unexpectedly appear, and even more so when they handcuff or otherwise restrain the student for transport. It's very upsetting to peers to witness this and may further stigmatize psychiatric treatment. Psychiatrists can be instrumental in consulting with public safety departments on campus *before* crises occur to explore options, such as sending out plainclothes officers to mental health emergencies, using unmarked cars to transport students, and establishing whether there are situations when a student can be safely transported without being restrained. If a counselor or residential staff member can accompany the student with the public safety officers, it often eases some of the student's anxiety.

Other considerations in working with student mental health emergencies include who to notify and when. Many students headed toward hospitalization agree to parental notification and give consent for notifying an adviser or a dean. It's always best to try to obtain consent, but in emergency situations, parents or deans can be notified without consent, if it seems in the student's best interest (or to protect the safety of others in the community). In the wake of the Virginia Tech massacre, the *Joint Guidance on the Application of the Family Educational Rights and Privacy Act (FERPA) and the Health Insurance Portability and Accountability Act of 1996 (HIPAA) to Student Health Records* was created to help clarify how FERPA and HIPAA intersect and how to balance privacy with health and safety.[5] These guidelines remind us that neither HIPAA nor FERPA prohibit disclosure of health information if the disclosure is deemed necessary to prevent or lessen threat of harm (and when disclosure is to people who can intervene to lessen the threat, including parents and school personnel).

The JED Foundation framework cautions against uniformly mandating or prohibiting notification, reminding us that this is a clinical decision we must make on a case-by-case basis. Consultation with peers or supervisors is helpful when considering notification without consent, if time allows. In the campus setting unique notification challenges arise, such as what to do about coaches or roommates of hospitalized students, who may become alarmed if a student seems to just disappear without explanation. Disclosure beyond family or deans is probably best left to the discretion of the dean (or family), except in situations when the safety of a specific person might be affected. The amount of information disclosed should be limited to the minimum necessary to protect safety.

It's important to reflect on what the student will gain by hospitalization. In my experience an ill-considered hospitalization can cause more harm than good, especially when, with the shrinking pool of inpatient beds, young students with mood disorders are hospitalized on wards with older, chronically mentally ill patients who exhibit psychotic or threatening behavior. Of course, sometimes hospitalization is the only way to ensure a student's safety, and sometimes it's the best way to achieve diagnostic clarity. Duration of hospitalization has dramatically decreased in recent years. In the large Virginia study of crisis interventions with college students, average length of stay when students were hospitalized was four days. In most cases that's time enough only to begin to stabilize a patient and ensure short-term safety, but not to provide meaningful treatment. That's why a vital part of managing emergencies is attending to the aftermath of hospitalization.

Assessing Violence

Many recent mass shootings, both on campus (such as Virginia Tech) and in other settings (the Aurora, Colorado, movie theater massacre) involve an emerging adult perpetrator who was enrolled in a university, or who had recently dropped out or was forced to leave. Although mass shootings are rare, other acts of violence and disruptive, threatening behaviors have been increasing on campus in recent years.[6] This means that all of us who work with students will be called on at some point to give an opinion about whether a student presents a significant threat to others.

From a clinical standpoint, psychiatrists can rely on their training in risk assessment to evaluate potential dangerousness in the context of a possible mental illness. We must pay particular attention to risk factors including (but not limited to) substance abuse and intoxication, psychotic symptoms (especially command hallucinations or other aggressive delusions), suicidal thoughts (many perpetrators of targeted violence are "suicidal without an escape plan"[7]), and a history of violence or self-harm. But psychiatric training, and the experience and evidence with which most clinicians working in college mental health are familiar, better prepares us to assess patients for risk to self than to others. Dangerous behaviors do not always occur in the context of mental health problems; we need to also recognize situations where law enforcement is the more appropriate route for evaluating a particular concern. If there are signs that an imminent threat is likely, or if the student is very agitated, the college counseling center is not the best place for evaluation; the psychiatrist can facilitate transport to an emergency department, for the safety of others at the counseling center as well as the student and others on campus.

Usually, evaluating dangerousness also relies on gathering and interpreting collateral information. In most cases, a student who has triggered community concern has exhibited troubling behaviors over time in a variety of contexts. All that information must be available to the clinician and must be reviewed. Even in the absence of a formal threat assessment team, psychiatrists called on to evaluate dangerousness need access to all the outside information that triggered evaluation, and they must have permission to speak with concerned others if necessary. There's a nascent field of research examining comprehensive, interdisciplinary approaches to creating safer campus communities, with a focus on behavioral intervention teams. Psychiatrists can be helpful collaborators in these approaches.

Threat Assessment versus Behavioral Intervention Teams

Interdisciplinary teams reviewed "students of concern" on college campuses even before the Virginia Tech shooting happened, but in the wake of that tragedy, the concept of more formalized, standing threat assessment teams evolved, was mandated in some states, and continues to change. There is growing recognition that we need a mechanism of early detection of individuals whose behavior is either alarming or threatening. In 2009, a group of people from various backgrounds, including attorneys, psychologists, student affairs personnel, and others from different universities across the country, formed an independent nonprofit organization, the National Behavioral Intervention Team Association (NaBITA), to act as a clearinghouse for best practices, training tools, and other supportive resources for creating safer campuses. (NaBITA provides an excellent whitepaper, *Threat Assessment in the Campus Setting*, at http://nabita .org/resources/threat-assessment-tools.)

The shift from "threat assessment" to "behavioral intervention" intends to convey that providing supportive resources and maintaining a philosophy that values caring campus communities is a better way to prevent aggressive acts than simply focusing on threats. "Threat assessment" also sounds threatening to all students and implies the potential for punitive action, perhaps making students more hesitant to report alarming behaviors. According to NaBITA, modern behavioral intervention teams provide a "proactive way to address the growing need in the college and university community for a centralized, coordinated, caring, developmental intervention for those in need prior to crisis."

Current threat assessment research has moved away from profiling—i.e., creating portraits of stereotypical aggressors—and from relying on written or verbal threats. Targeted campus violence is often a perfect storm of a potential attacker, the attacker's history of stressful events, a current situation that acts as a trigger, and targets; usually a host of behaviors and planning lead up to the violence.[8] For these reasons, neither profiling nor direct communication of threats is a very effective predictor. Because campuses are open communities, many different people may have concerns about the same student, but unless there is a centralized method for gathering everyone's concerns and evaluating these in context, intervention is difficult. At Duke we've created a safety net called DukeReach, which allows anyone in the university community to report concerns (anonymously or not) about a student's behavior to one phone number (or Web site). This centralized reporting system links with, and is just one aspect of, an effective behavioral intervention team.

A whitepaper recently prepared by the National Center of Higher Education Risk Management (NCHERM) outlines 12 elements of current best practices for behavioral intervention teams. These are listed in table 17.1.

If a student does trigger concerns about becoming violent, and is in our clinical opinion also showing signs of a psychiatric illness, then hospitalization is a good option. It's particularly important to remember that if a student is placed on mandatory leave because of mental illness with the potential for violence (to self as well as others), that student needs a well-thought-out treatment plan. Students who go on leave for mental health reasons without a treatment plan in place seem particularly vulnerable to bad outcomes, although there is little systematic evidence to prove this.

Psychiatrist's Role during Hospitalization and in Discharge Planning

There are no evidence-based recommendations for the best way a campus or community psychiatrist can collaborate with inpatient teams when a student is hospitalized, and practices vary widely, often depending on the treatment model of the outpatient provider. Because many counseling centers historically and by necessity are brief treatment centers, hospitalization often suggests that a student will need, upon discharge, a higher level of care than that afforded by

Table 17.1   NCHERM best practices for behavioral intervention teams

1. Modern behavioral intervention teams use formalized protocols of explicit engagement techniques and strategies.
2. Modern behavioral intervention teams see their role as nominally to address threat, and primarily to support and provide resources to students.
3. Modern behavioral intervention teams utilize mandated psychological assessment.
4. Modern behavioral intervention teams have the authority to invoke involuntary medical or psychological withdrawal policies.
5. Modern behavioral intervention teams are undergirded by sophisticated threat assessment capacity, beyond law enforcement and psychological assessment tools.
6. Modern behavioral intervention teams use risk rubrics to classify threats.
7. Modern behavioral intervention teams foster a comprehensive reporting culture within the institution.
8. Modern behavioral intervention teams train and educate the community on what to report and how.
9. Modern behavioral intervention teams are technologically advanced and supported by comprehensive databases that allow the team to have a longitudinal view of a student's behavior patterns and trends.
10. Modern behavioral intervention teams focus not only on student-based risks but on faculty and staff as well.
11. Modern behavioral intervention teams intentionally integrate with campus risk management programs and risk mitigation strategies.
12. Modern behavioral intervention teams have a mechanism for "minding the gap."

Source: Sokolow, B. A., & Lewis, W. S. (2009). *2nd generation behavioral intervention best practices.* NCHERM whitepaper, www.ncherm.org/2009NCHERMwhitepaper.pdf.

the counseling center. This varies across universities and case by case. If for financial or logistical reasons, no other psychiatrists are available to take care of the student, then treatment within the counseling center may be the best option. Obviously, psychiatrists in private practice have much greater latitude to work with students regardless of the intensity and duration of their needs.

Even if we will not be providing the discharge care of a student we've treated, unless we saw her for only a one-session emergency evaluation, it is good care to check in with the student during the hospitalization or in a bridge appointment after, to bring our work to a helpful conclusion and explain why a referral is necessary when that's the case. It's also important to ensure that the student actually follows through with the plan for referral. If referring a student after hospital discharge, I ask for permission to contact the clinician and ask that clinician to confirm that the student has kept her appointment. If a hospital or emergency department refers a student back to us for a post-discharge appointment, we notify the referring clinician if the student fails to keep that appointment, so the clinician can follow up with the student.

I agree with the JED Foundation framework's recommendation that "discharge planning should begin at the time of admission." Because academic semesters move at a rapid pace, having a good treatment plan in place early is critical to the student's chances of finishing out the semester after a hospitalization, or for facilitating a medical leave when that's needed. The counseling center psychiatrist is often the expert on university mental health referral resources in the larger local community and as such can be extremely helpful to the inpatient team. Again, the level of involvement depends on specific laws and the relationship between a hospital and a counseling center. If the counseling center is part of a campus-wide integrated medical system, as is the case at Duke, then under HIPAA the emergency department can notify the counseling center each time a student is psychiatrically evaluated, which greatly facilitates follow-up care.

An important consideration for every hospitalized student is whether the student might benefit from—or in some cases, absolutely need—a medical leave of absence. It's helpful to remind students, families, and inpatient teams that this is an option. Sometimes less extreme accommodations can help a student stay in school while getting better, such as withdrawing from a single class, or taking incompletes in one or more classes. Psychiatrists and other mental health providers are invaluable consultants in this process, but the ultimate decision to cut back on academic load or to withdraw rests with the student and the dean. Sometimes the student and dean or others involved in the student's care disagree about whether a leave is necessary. Many universities have crafted policies for involuntary leave, outlining the situations in which a school can mandate time off if deans are concerned that a student cannot safely function in the university community.

It's crucial that universities clearly communicate expectations for treatment to the student who goes on medical leave. In Virginia, nearly 50% of public colleges and 91% of private colleges have procedures for initiating mandated leave for mental health reasons, and these almost always specify requirements for documentation of adherence to recommended treatment if students pursue readmission.

If a student's readmission to the university will be contingent on mental health treatment during leave, this should be specified *before* the leave. Ideally, every student going on leave for psychological reasons should receive the same written guidelines from the school, but not all schools have created such guidelines. At the least, the university should provide the student with a clear written summary of the expectations for treatment; psychiatrists are often asked to spell these out.

Sometimes, psychiatrists are asked to review the treatment of a student returning from leave, or to evaluate the student (in addition to reviewing records of treatment) to determine readiness for return. These can be complex requests, since the student's goals and the university's may differ, creating a potential conflict of interest for the psychiatrist. The decision to readmit is always the school's. At many universities the policy is for the dean to consult with the director of the counseling service or the director's designee, allowing for a more uniform review process.

A Note of Caution about the Anxious Campus

Campus mass shootings are terrifying, and campus suicides are extremely upsetting; in our zeal to develop mechanisms to minimize risk, we can overreact. As we create safety webs and behavioral intervention teams and work to educate university communities about our collective role in maintaining vigilance to certain behavioral red flags, it's critical to match the intervention strategy we employ to the level of risk we've identified. Otherwise, we might force to clinical attention students whose behaviors are not dangerous, and inadvertently cause *them* emotional harm. As campuses become increasingly diverse, conflicts may arise from differences in cultural interpretations of behavior, and handling these requires both knowledge and sensitivity. One example is the vignette below:

> Campus safety officers bring Babafemi, a 20-year-old freshman from Nigeria, to a counseling center evaluation after two hallmates reported concerns about his behavior. A female student complained that he'd followed her around at a party, making her uncomfortable and trailing her into the women's bathroom. A male student reported an altercation in which Babafemi slapped a wall, cursed, and muttered, "You'll be sorry." When the resident adviser confronted him, Babafemi threw up his hands and then "took off" without discussing the situation. She called campus safety to find him and do a wellness check. When he became "belligerent" at their questions, they asked if he'd like to go to the counseling center, and reportedly he agreed.

Babafemi is a muscular young man who speaks heavily accented English, makes little eye contact initially, and hangs his head. He seems confused about the nature of the center and the evaluation, thinking he's "in trouble" even though he "didn't do anything." He admits he didn't understand exactly what the "police" were asking him, so he agreed to go wherever they said he had to. When the nature of the session is explained to him, he relaxes and becomes nearly tearful.

He admits that these first five months of college in the United States have been more challenging than he'd expected. He was particularly lonely over winter break, since he couldn't afford to go home and had to move into the only dorm remaining open for international students. He began second semester with the renewed goal of making American friends, but his efforts have been unfruitful. He got drunk at the party at which he followed the girl into the bathroom and felt extremely ashamed after. When he went to apologize to her the next day, she refused to talk to him, and she seemed afraid of him. Just after that encounter, he ran into a group of male students in the common room. He tried to join them but was told it was a private session for fraternity members only and was asked to leave. Some of the students snickered at his name, which insulted him. One joked, "What kind of a name is that for a man?" He did slap the wall and curse but maintains that he had no plan or intent to fight any of the other students; he is aghast that "you'll be sorry" was taken to mean he'd ever physically hurt them. He was terrified when the public safety officers, whom he took for city police, appeared; he trembles and becomes tearful discussing how he thought he was being arrested and didn't understand why. He denies any history of violence, including relationship violence.

Applying NaBITA's model of classifying risk and matching intervention tools to risk as assessed, the scenario above suggests a mild to moderate level of risk (concerning behaviors, a possible threat, which is vague and indirect, unclear level of student distress). Examples of mild- to moderate-level interventions include confrontation by the RA, conflict management or mediation, a possible behavioral contract, or, depending on how these progress, possible referral for psychological evaluation if the student's distress escalates during conflict resolution. But Babafemi took off before the less severe interventions could be attempted, which might signal greater emotional distress, or simply a lack of understanding, perhaps based on cultural differences, of what was expected of him in that moment. The RA activated public safety, who under ideal circumstances would have brought the student back to the dorm for a discussion. Instead, through a miscommunication, the student was transported to an evaluation, which in the NaBITA rubric is a recommended intervention for elevated to severe risk. International students, or other students whose English language skills are limited, are especially vulnerable to miscommunications and potentially escalated responses to fairly age-normative conflicts.

> Babafemi agrees to a follow-up visit in two weeks. At that session he reports difficulty sleeping and some nightmares in which he is arrested and taken to jail. He has been keeping to himself for fear of saying or doing something that will upset another student and is entirely avoiding parties. He reports an apathetic or numb mood. He's had trouble concentrating, and his grades have declined slightly, but he denies self-harm or violent thoughts. He's been reconsidering whether it was a good idea to pursue college in the United States, so far from his family, but he doesn't want to disappoint his family by cutting short his studies.

This vignette illustrates the costs of hypervigilance with regard to safety on campus. In this case there was no clear danger to the community, but rather an absence of data about a potential threat. Activating an escalated response may have caused this student to have an adjustment reaction, or even acute traumatic stress; he is now at some risk of dropping out of the university. There are examples in the literature of colleges reacting to potentially suicidal students by locking them out of their dorm and placing them on mandatory leave before their psychiatric evaluation is even complete[9]—a clear over-reaction to the potential for self-harm. It's important to resist reacting to the anxiety caused by well-publicized acts of violence with over-reactions to student conflicts. Interactions between students—and especially between students from differing backgrounds—can become quite complex, and interventions require evidence-based information and cultural sensitivity along with a continual balancing of the benefits and risks to a given individual against those to the community.

Impulse Control Problems, Behavioral Addictions, and Other Problematic Behaviors

Jim, a 22-year old Caucasian senior student from Texas, comes in at the suggestion of his fiancée, Allie. She is concerned that he has been spending too much time online, and his secretive habits regarding his computer use make her worry that he is viewing pornography. He explains that although he occasionally uses online porn, most of his time online is spent gambling. He gambles several times a week, spending a few hours total each week, and has long since exceeded his monthly income. He is secretive because he knows his fiancée would disapprove, but he made nearly $5,000 at the beginning of the year, which financed not only part of his final year of college but also much of their courtship. In the past two months his luck has turned, and he's lost nearly $2,000. He's borrowed money from friends and, more recently, from his mother, to whom he lied about why he needed the money. He sometimes feels out of control of his gambling but is sure once he wins and can repay his debts, he can stop.

Nineteen-year old Caucasian sophomore Olivia comes in complaining of insomnia and stress. She's shy and has had a tough adjustment to college, but she settled in with a few friends first year. Now her friends have rushed a sorority, and she no longer feels welcome in their circle but has made no new friends. During the course of her evaluation for anxiety, the clinician asks about the baseball cap she wears tightly covering her head. She flushes and explains she has bald patches where she's been pulling out her hair. This has been a long-standing problem, which greatly embarrasses her and is one of the reasons she requested a single dorm room. She's never before discussed it with a health care provider, and as she does, she begins to cry.

Some impulse control problems were characterized in the psychiatric literature long ago, and others are newer, related to novel technologies that are pervasive in our present-day society. And there's been debate around classification of certain problematic behaviors. Are they addictions? Are they impulse control disorders? Some of these answers will no doubt come once we better understand the neurobiological mechanisms underlying repetitive behaviors that get people into trouble. Regardless, a significant number of college students find their lives disrupted by problematic behavior that is not necessarily part of their presenting concern for counseling, but which causes enough distress and impairment that it's important to assess and address in the course of mental health treatment.

Several problematic behaviors, including trichotillomania (pathological hair pulling), skin-picking (excoriation disorder), and hoarding, have been added or reclassified in DSM-5, grouped with obsessive-compulsive disorder to reflect a growing understanding of these conditions' relatedness to one another. Gambling disorder has been added to the substance-related disorders section. Kleptomania is classified with disruptive, impulse control, and conduct disorders. Although these groupings suggest some differences between these problematic behaviors, and researchers are trying to better understand the neurobiological underpinnings and phenomenological presentations, from a clinical standpoint all these problems involve failure to suppress the urge or temptation to perform an action that has harmful consequences to the person or to others.[1] People experience tension before the repetitive act and sometimes craving. They experience relief or pleasure during the act. With repeated engagement in the act, however, there's diminished pleasure or relief and a sense of loss of control, leading to an increase in the behavior in an attempt to recapture the pleasure. People may try to cut back unsuccessfully. Over time these behaviors cause impaired functioning in work, school, and social settings.

Although research is limited (in part because not all of these problems have clear diagnostic definitions), one study of nearly 800 college students at two midwestern colleges found that impulse control problems are common, affecting as many as one in ten.[2] Most common were trichotillomania and compulsive sexual behavior. There are some gender differences. Male students more frequently had problems with pathological gambling and compulsive sexual behavior, and female students with compulsive buying. Kleptomania was least commonly observed.

There are high rates of comorbidity between pathological gambling, kleptomania, compulsive sexual behavior, Internet addiction, and substance addictions. There may be a shared neurobiological problem that leads to both substance addiction and impulse control problems in another area. Some resist labeling these other problematic behaviors as separate disorders, arguing that they may simply be different manifestations of the same underlying disease process, such as a personality disorder or a substance addiction. However, in working with college students it is helpful to be aware of and address some of these more common impulse control problems as part of their evaluation and treatment.

Internet "Addiction"?

With the rise in importance of the Internet in academic communities, more and more students (and faculty) are spending significant amounts of time online. For some students, excessive use begins to take on the characteristics of a behavioral addiction. Because currently there aren't defined criteria, it's difficult to diagnose or estimate prevalence rates with consistency, but problematic Internet use generally has the following four components. It is excessive, with people often losing a sense of time and neglecting other drives; it causes withdrawal (unpleasant tension or craving) when computers are unavailable; there's tolerance, leading to increased use over time or to preoccupation with increasingly sophisticated or expensive computer equipment; and it causes negative consequences, including poor academic performance, social isolation, and significant fatigue.[3] In other countries there have been instances of young men neglecting eating or other basic self-care, to the point of physical danger—and even death—because of online activities. According to the DSM-5, the Chinese government has defined Internet gaming as an "addiction" and set up a treatment system.

Excessive online time seems to fall into one of at least three categories: gaming, cybersex, or e-mail and messaging. Much of the research on Internet addiction has been carried out in Europe and Asia and finds high rates of comorbidity with mood, anxiety disorders—especially social and generalized anxiety—and ADHD among youth.

Because some reports suggest that as many as 13% of undergraduates suffer from Internet addiction, one research group in Taiwan developed diagnostic criteria and a screening tool specifically for college students.[4] In their study, as in others, Internet-addicted students were more likely to be male and more likely to participate in online gaming than nonaddicted students. Another large study of Turkish college students found that over 12% of the men, compared to only 5.5% of the women, were problematic Internet users, and that men and women differed in their patterns of use.[5] Men more often spent time online playing games, while women spent more time in chat rooms and messaging. Among these Turkish students, those with the highest scores on an instrument screening for Internet addiction also had the highest scores on a measure of dissociative symptoms, the Dissociative Experiences Scale (DES). This suggests that those who excessively use the Internet are also more frequently dissociating. Students with a dissociative disorder most frequently used the Internet for messaging or chat rooms. Various studies also report what is echoed in our students' complaints: that excessive Internet use leads to lost productivity in academic work, a sense of lost time, interpersonal problems, and an increased sense of loneliness. Sleep disruption and fatigue are other common sequelae.

Internet gaming disorder is included in section 3 of the DSM-5 as a condition recommended for further study (see table 18.1). Given the high incidence of problematic Internet use among college students, who increasingly *must* spend time online to do their schoolwork, it is important to assess Internet use among students presenting with various psychiatric symptoms, and to address it in our treatment planning. Although empirical evidence on effective treatments is limited, some early studies suggest that various forms of psychotherapy, including group and individual CBT; motivational interviewing; reality therapy; and a multimodal treatment approach lead to significant improvement.[6] Case reports and an open-label followed by double-blind discontinuation study of SSRI pharmacological treatment likewise look promising. Treating comorbid depression and anxiety may improve Internet addiction as well. At the very least, problem solving with students about ways to reduce Internet use when they view it as problematic, and providing psychoeducation about ways it can interfere with sleep and circadian rhythms, is a critical part of a holistic treatment approach, while we await more research-guided recommendations. Sometimes something as simple as recommending software that disables Inter-

Table 18.1   Proposed criteria for Internet gaming disorder in DSM-5

Persistent and recurrent use of the Internet to engage in games, often with other players, leading to clinically significant impairment or distress as indicated by five (or more) of the following in a 12-month period:

1. Preoccupation with Internet games (the individual thinks about previous gaming activity or anticipates playing the next game; Internet gaming becomes the dominant activity in daily life).
2. Withdrawal symptoms when Internet gaming is taken away (these symptoms are typically described as irritability, anxiety, or sadness, but there are no physical signs of pharmacological withdrawal).
3. Tolerance—the need to spend increasing amounts of time in Internet games.
4. Unsuccessful attempts to control participation in Internet games.
5. Loss of interest in previous hobbies and entertainment as a result of, and with the exception of, Internet games.
6. Continued excessive use of Internet games despite knowledge of psychosocial problems.
7. Has deceived family members, therapists, or others regarding the amount of Internet gaming.
8. Use of Internet games to escape or relieve a negative mood (e.g., feelings of helplessness, guilt, anxiety).
9. Has jeopardized or lost a significant relationship, job, or educational or career opportunity because of participation in Internet games.

Source: From American Psychiatric Association. (2013). *Diagnostic and statistical manual of mental disorders,* 5th ed. (DSM-5). Washington, D.C.: American Psychiatric Association.

Note: Only nongambling Internet games are included in this disorder. Use of the Internet for required activities in a business or profession is not included; nor is the disorder intended to include other recreational or social Internet use. Similarly, sexual Internet sites are excluded. Specifying current severity: Internet gaming disorder can be mild, moderate, or severe, depending on the degree of disruption of normal activities. Individuals with less severe Internet gaming disorder may exhibit fewer symptoms and less disruption of their lives. Those with severe Internet gaming disorder will have more hours spent on the computer and more significant loss of relationships or career or school opportunities.

net access for a specified time (programs such as Self-Control or Freedom, some available free of charge online) can help a student focus on school assignments rather than spiral into cycles of distraction and self-recrimination.

In the first vignette above, Jim is spending large amounts of time online, though he seems to view it as less of a problem than does his fiancée. The bulk of his time is spent gambling. Problematic gambling can affect students both online and in other contexts.

Pathological Gambling

Pathological gambling, or a recurrent and persistent pattern of gambling behavior that leads to significant psychosocial and financial problems, occurs in 0.5 to 1.0% of community samples when based on diagnostic rather than screening assessment.[7] Self-report screening inventories find much higher rates of problematic gambling. One study using a self-rated screening instrument found a rate of about 0.6% among college students, but many surveys find higher rates, ranging from 2.9% to over 9%, the latter in athletes.[8] Some studies suggest that as many as one in six college athletes has a gambling problem and that certain groups are particularly vulnerable. In general men are affected more than women. Among athletes, older students, students from minority racial groups, and those who are members of a fraternity or sorority have the highest risk of pathological gambling.[9] Compared with recreational gamblers or nongambling students, college students in the pathological gambling category have more academic problems and are greater risk takers, more likely to engage in heavier alcohol and illicit drug use and unprotected sex.[10] In rare instances students have murdered bookies and committed suicide because of gambling debt.[11]

When gambling is considered on a continuum, *problematic* gambling occurs at even higher rates among college students and appears to be on the rise. Gambling activities range from casino gambling to card games and betting on sporting events. Online gambling has increased on campuses, prompting the National Association of Student Personnel Administrators to form a gambling task force and leading many universities to begin gambling education and intervention programs.[12] In recognition of many shared phenomenological as well as neurobiological features between pathological gambling and substance abuse, in DSM-5 pathological gambling was moved from the impulse control disorders category into the "Substance-Related and Addictive Disorders" section and dubbed gambling disorder (see table 18.2).

Screening instruments, such as the South Oaks Gambling Screen (SOGS), can help identify whether a student like Jim falls into a category of concerning gambling. He already presents several higher-risk behavioral indicators, based on those found in a study of gambling in college students: gambling more than once a month, spending more than two hours per month on gambling, and risking more than 10% of his monthly income.[13] Because of high comorbidity between pathological gambling and substance abuse, he should have a full substance use assessment. His evaluation should also include questions about legal difficulties.

Many people with pathological gambling recover without formal treatment

Table 18.2   Diagnostic criteria for gambling disorder in DSM-5

A. Persistent and recurrent problematic gambling behavior leading to clinically signifi-
    cant impairment or distress, as indicated by the individual exhibiting four (or more) of
    the following in a 12-month period:
    1. Needs to gamble with increasing amounts of money in order to achieve the desired
        excitement.
    2. Is restless or irritable when attempting to cut down or stop gambling.
    3. Has made repeated unsuccessful efforts to control, cut back, or stop gambling.
    4. Is often preoccupied with gambling (e.g., having persistent thoughts of reliving past
        gambling experiences, handicapping or planning the next venture, or thinking of
        ways to get money with which to gamble).
    5. Often gambles when feeling distressed (e.g., helpless, guilty, anxious, depressed).
    6. After losing money gambling, often returns another day to get even ("chasing" one's
        losses).
    7. Lies to conceal the extent of involvement with gambling.
    8. Has jeopardized or lost a significant relationship, job, or educational or career
        opportunity because of gambling.
    9. Relies on others to provide money to relieve desperate financial situations caused
        by gambling.
B. The gambling behavior is not better explained by a manic episode.

Source: From American Psychiatric Association. (2013). *Diagnostic and statistical manual of mental
disorders,* 5th ed. (DSM-5). Washington, D.C.: American Psychiatric Association.

or intervention, but for college students, the stakes of not addressing the problem may be high. For example, significant debts may lead students to break the
law or to take on jobs that interfere with classwork, jeopardizing their ability
to remain in or graduate from college. In Jim's case, it is already straining his
relationships and may put his upcoming marriage at risk. Some suggest that
the residential college environment partially insulates students from the negative consequences of gambling, since they have food, housing, and families or
friends who can help them financially. Jim, as a senior, may face particularly
difficult circumstances in the next year if he doesn't address his gambling before graduation. Although this hasn't been systematically studied yet, early intervention may keep some students from significant deterioration later in life.

Psychosocial treatments such as CBT, often modified from a substance
abuse model, and brief motivational therapy have shown efficacy for treating
pathological gambling in randomized controlled trials. Data from randomized, placebo-controlled trials of SSRIs have been mixed. The most promising
pharmacological agents are the opioid receptor antagonists naltrexone and
nalmefene.[14]

Trichotillomania and Other Body-Focused Repetitive Behaviors

Recurrent pulling out of one's own hair, leading to hair loss, is more common among college students than previously thought. As with some of the other less-studied problems in this chapter, the criteria for diagnosis are in the midst of modification as new research emerges about genetics, neurobiology, and epidemiology. DSM-5 has reclassified the diagnosis from an impulse control disorder to an obsessive-compulsive spectrum problem. Studies that used different definitions make it difficult to find accurate prevalence rates, but existing studies of problematic hair pulling in college students report prevalence of between 1% and 13.3%.[15] More recently it's become clear that there are different subtypes of hair pulling, and that the behavior is not always accompanied by the rising sense of tension prior to the act and relief after that was previously required for diagnosis (see table 18.3). Childhood onset hair pulling begins by age 8 and often spontaneously remits. Adolescent onset may persist, and emerging adults with hair pulling may fall into the three-quarters of people who pull automatically, without awareness, or the one-quarter who are more focused, and feel a compulsion to pull.[16] There is, of course, overlap between these two groups. The distinction likely has implications for best treatment approaches. Though traditionally considered a disorder mainly of women, trichotillomania studies in college samples show a fairly high proportion of affected male students as well. One study of 2,500 college students found a 3.4% lifetime prevalence rate for women and 1.5% for men.[17]

Olivia's avoidance of social activities, as described in the vignette above, is a common result of trichotillomania and may also signal a comorbid anxiety disorder. Mood and anxiety diagnoses, OCD, and eating disorders all occur at much higher rates in people with significant hair pulling. Most commonly af-

Table 18.3   Diagnostic criteria for trichotillomania (hair-pulling disorder) in DSM-5

A. Recurrent pulling out of one's hair, resulting in hair loss.
B. Repeated attempts to decrease or stop hair pulling.
C. The hair pulling causes clinically significant distress or impairment in social, occupational, or other important areas of functioning.
D. The hair pulling or hair loss is not attributable to a general medical condition (e.g., a dermatological condition).
E. The hair pulling is not better explained by the symptoms of another mental disorder (e.g., attempts to improve a perceived defect or flaw in appearance in body dysmorphic disorder).

Source: From American Psychiatric Association. (2013). *Diagnostic and statistical manual of mental disorders,* 5th ed. (DSM-5). Washington, D.C.: American Psychiatric Association.

Table 18.4   Diagnostic criteria for excoriation (skin-picking) disorder in DSM-5

A. Recurrent skin picking resulting in skin lesions.
B. Repeated attempts to decrease or stop skin picking.
C. The skin picking causes clinically significant distress or impairment in social, occupational, or other important areas of functioning.
D. The skin picking is not attributable to the direct physiological effects of a substance (e.g., cocaine) or another medical condition (e.g., scabies).
E. The skin picking is not better explained by symptoms of another mental disorder (e.g., delusions or tactile hallucinations in a psychotic disorder, attempts to improve a perceived defect or flaw in appearance in body dysmorphic disorder, stereotypies in stereotypic movement disorder, or intention to harm oneself in nonsuicidal self-injury).

Source: From American Psychiatric Association. (2013). *Diagnostic and statistical manual of mental disorders,* 5th ed. (DSM-5). Washington, D.C.: American Psychiatric Association.

fected is the scalp, but students also pull eyebrows, eyelashes, or hair elsewhere on the body, including pubic hair.

Students who pull hair also more frequently engage in other body-focused repetitive behaviors, such as skin picking or nail biting. Of these two, more problematic is skin picking, or repetitively touching blemishes or skin irregularities until there is bleeding or tissue damage. Students usually use their fingers to pick but may also use objects, such as tweezers. Most are highly embarrassed by their behavior. Although skin picking is common to some extent in most people, including college students, self-injurious skin picking affects about 4% of college students and is likely even more common in counseling center populations because of high comorbidity with OCD and other anxiety disorders.[18] Problematic skin picking, compared to the more benign varieties, occupies more of the person's time, causes distress, defies attempts to cut back, and can cause medically significant problems. In recognition of all this, excoriation disorder is listed as a new disorder in the "Obsessive-Compulsive and Related Disorders" section (see table 18.4).

Olivia's evaluation should include careful screening for anxiety disorders, symptoms of a tic disorder, and eating and body image concerns. One well-validated instrument that can both assess symptoms of hair pulling and monitor treatment response is the Massachusetts General Hospital (MGH) Hair-pulling Scale, available online. There is a similar MGH Skin-Picking Scale.

If other anxiety or mood problems surface during Olivia's evaluation, treating these may improve the hair pulling. Psychoeducation about the biological nature of hair-pulling disorder and the existence of effective treatments can help diminish Olivia's sense of shame. It's important not to ask to assess the affected hair loss site before forming a good therapeutic alliance.[19] The attempt to diminish shame and stigma associated with the diagnosis was part of the discussion behind changing the name of the disorder in DSM-5, from trichotillomania to skin-picking disorder. However, both terms are now in use.

There's more evidence supporting psychotherapeutic rather than psychopharmacologic approaches to the treatment of hair pulling, though medication may also help. Behavioral therapy with a habit-reversal component is most strongly supported by existing evidence.[20] Cognitive behavioral therapies that incorporate other techniques, including self-monitoring, relaxation, and cognitive restructuring, also help. Randomized controlled medication trials have had mixed results, but clomipramine did seem effective in one such trial.[21] Open-label studies and some randomized controlled trials suggest that SSRIs may be beneficial. Certainly if there is comorbid depression or anxiety, antidepressant treatment with an SSRI is a good place to start, preferably in combination with behavioral therapy. One small double-blind placebo-controlled trial suggested efficacy of the amino acid N-acetylcysteine, in doses of 1200–2400 milligrams per day.[22] Other case reports and open-label studies also find N-acetylcysteine promising for the treatment of impulse control problems as well as addictions, including pathological gambling and skin picking. Pathological skin picking may also respond to SSRI treatment, as one double-blind trial of fluoxetine and several other open-label trials suggest.[23]

CHAPTER 19

The Nontraditional Student

Maria, a married Hispanic woman who returned to college this year, has to reschedule her initial assessment appointment twice before explaining to the front desk that she's had trouble arranging childcare; she is then invited to bring her child with her, and an administrative staff member volunteers to watch the four-year-old while Maria is evaluated. A professor referred 25-year-old Maria to counseling after Maria failed to turn in several papers on time and burst into tears about her subsequent grades. Maria admits she's felt overwhelmed since starting the semester, often feels behind, and wonders if she's as capable as her younger peers, who seem to breeze through their classes.

Today's university campus is significantly more diverse than that of a generation ago, and this diversity includes greater numbers of students who don't fit the traditional undergraduate stereotype of young, single, and financially dependent on their parents. Definitions of nontraditional vary from those based solely on age to broader ones that take into account marital status, other dependents, employment status, and other factors, including military service. Students aged 24 and older accounted for 28% of the college population in 1970, but for 44% in 2001.[1] By the mid-nineties, 21% of undergraduates had dependents other than a spouse, and 27% worked full time.

Women over 25 are the fastest-growing population in higher education institutions, and they frequently have to juggle multiple roles—including parenting—which can lead to emotional adversity.[2] At the same time, research suggests that some students actually benefit from having multiple roles. Understanding differences in developmental stages between nontraditional and traditional students as well as within groups of nontraditional students can help us work more effectively with them when they present for psychiatric care. And because the absence of psychological distress is apparently the best predictor of retention for nontraditional students, good psychiatric care will allow more of these students to meet their educational goals.

Unfortunately, little data exist on the psychiatric needs of these groups. Existing research on adjustment of nontraditional students focuses more on women than on men, and more on academic than on psychological issues. One study that compared nontraditional to traditional students found that the nontraditional group valued their academic work more but actually attended classes less; this study did not replicate an earlier finding that nontraditional students were more anxious about schoolwork.[3] The authors hypothesized that the added responsibilities outside of school, and satisfaction in other roles, allowed the older students to have a more complex self-image and be less worried about schoolwork. However, individual differences obviously greatly affect this. For students like Maria, returning to school as a mother, studies suggest that secure attachment, a sense of self-efficacy both as student and as parent, and social support best protect against psychological distress when stressors mount.[4] It's important, therefore, to understand Maria's relationships with her husband and other family members as well as her past experiences as a student.

Maria and her husband moved away from extended family so that she could pursue her education at her dream school. Her husband works full time to support them and is unable to help much with childcare responsibilities, such as taking time off when their daughter is ill. Maria has thus had to miss class multiple times, but she notes that her younger peers miss even more class yet seem less affected by it. Maria's parents are Mexican, and she was raised in Texas. They've had a hard time understanding why she would choose a school in another state, so far from the family. When she complains about her difficulties in phone calls home, her mother reminds her that life would have been easier had she stayed close by.

Compared to traditional undergraduates and to nontraditional male students, nontraditional female students are more likely to lack confidence in their ability to be a student,[5] which affects performance. They also spend less time in social or extracurricular campus activities than their traditional-aged peers, and thus do not often know their classmates well. This may make them less inclined to ask to share notes from missed classes, for example. It can also exacerbate feelings of isolation when other support systems are not in place. In Maria's case, moving far away from her family and the conflicts this generated can make her more vulnerable to the stresses of the transition. She may also be defying cultural norms in moving away from her family. Normalizing this in the course of working with her, while also exploring ways she can realistically expand her social network, are important interventions.

Nontraditional students of both genders report higher intrinsic motivation to learn—greater curiosity, interest in the work, learning as an end in itself—than traditional undergraduates, but they are equally extrinsically motivated—by grades or outcome.[6] Some researchers find that undue emphasis on grades or other extrinsic factors creates more problems for older students and suggest that validating older students' academic competence, encouraging autonomy, and treating them as active partners in learning all lead to better outcomes for them. Thus therapy with a student facing academic challenges, as Maria is, might focus on ways she can advocate for herself with her professors and advisers, such as requesting more and earlier feedback on her work. With permission we might also consult with her professors and share some of these data.

The emphasis in therapeutic work with nontraditional students is usually different than with younger students. Older students tend to drink and party less. They worry less about social interactions. They may already be better at self-care, including getting regular sleep and exercise, though nontraditional women get less physical exercise than their male peers.[7] But because they are in college, they sometimes face issues around separation-individuation (as Maria demonstrates) and identity development. They also experience barriers to engaging in their education, including caring for children, employment, and living off campus and having to navigate transportation to attend class. Practical solutions to address these needs, such as childcare and flexible scheduling when possible, allow these students to engage in treatment as well as modeling for them how to negotiate these challenges in other areas of their lives.

No clear evidence suggests that nontraditional students suffer depression or anxiety at higher rates than traditional students. Maria should be fully evaluated in the same way that younger undergraduates would be. One study at the University of Utah looked at risk factors for suicide among students, a large portion of whom would be considered nontraditional due to older age, living off campus, and being married. The researchers found that living off campus was a risk factor, as were a history of emotional abuse or assault, or identifying as not heterosexual; employment seemed to reduce risk.[8] Although the study authors emphasized that the student body at the University of Utah has several unique characteristics that may preclude their findings from generalizing to other student populations, other research has identified isolation, LGBT status, and a history of abuse as contributing to increased risk of self-harm, so non-traditional students who have one or more of these characteristics should trigger an especially careful evaluation for suicidal thoughts.

Veterans on Campus

Marcus is a 24-year-old Caucasian freshman from Louisiana who comes in complaining of difficulty sleeping, nightmares, and daytime fatigue. He is also easily irritated with his classmates, who all seem juvenile to him. Although he worries about grades, their worries seem excessive and their concerns with fraternity rush and athletics seem trivial. He was deployed in Afghanistan and Iraq and was involved in combat during his second deployment. He'd originally started college before the second deployment but was pulled from his first semester when a service need arose. He would like to "just forget about all that and have a chance to be a regular college student now."

As millions of troops return from protracted wars in the Middle East, the numbers of student veterans in college have grown and will likely continue to do so. Due to the post-9/11 GI bill, colleges are seeing the highest numbers of student veterans since World War II. In 2009 34, 393 veterans were receiving GI bill benefits, and in 2011 that mushroomed to more than a half million.[9] According to the Department of Defense, the decade of combat has led to increasing rates of psychological problems for service members, including high rates of PTSD, depression, suicide, and substance abuse.[10] Veterans navigating the transition to college are not immune from this elevated risk and may have the additional stressors of being in a new environment and of feeling out of sync with peers due to age and experience. They also face academic challenges that differ from the sorts of challenges they encountered in the military; as is the case for Marcus, years may have elapsed between graduation from high school and matriculation in college, during which academic knowledge and skills have likely eroded. And unlike veterans who entered college after World War II, who almost all graduated, current veterans face drop-out rates as high as 88% in addition to isolation on campus.[11]

One large survey study of a national sample of student veterans found them plagued by frequent and severe psychological symptoms, including suicidal thoughts and attempts.[12] These far outpaced the rates in general college student sample surveys, such as the American College Health Association's National College Health Assessment. Among the 525 student veterans who completed a 34-item survey, which included the PHQ-9, the GAD-7, the Insomnia-Severity Index-Abbreviated, and a measure of PTSD symptoms, almost 35% experienced "severe anxiety," 23.7% reported "severe depression," and over 45% experienced significant PTSD symptoms.[13] Nearly 50% of these students had experienced suicidal thoughts, 20% with a plan. More than 10% experienced suicidal thoughts "often or very often," and 7.7% had made a suicide attempt. These alarmingly elevated numbers suggest an urgent need for increased vigilance and perhaps specialized training for all of us who work with student veterans, to ensure we're meeting the needs of these men and women who served our country, often at great personal cost.

Research on veterans returning from the operations in Afghanistan and Iraq finds that younger age in active duty increases the risk of PTSD, as do multiple deployments, number of high combat experiences, and being wounded in combat.[14] Thus Marcus's evaluation must include questions about injuries, including exposure to explosions. Furthermore, alcohol, marijuana, and tobacco use are common among returning veterans, and younger veterans are more likely to experience new-onset binge drinking after return from deployment.[15] Given that the college environment already puts emerging adults at increased risk for binge drinking, we must remain alert to the particular vulnerability of student veterans to substance abuse.

The differential diagnosis for a student like Marcus is broad. When a veteran complains of nightmares, he obviously must be screened for PTSD, but in fact all student veterans presenting for mental health care should be screened for PTSD given its high incidence among returning troops and its significant morbidity. Some researchers recommend broad screenings of nonclinical student veteran populations during orientation or other points early in the transition to college. PTSD appears to increase the risk of suicide even when other factors, such as depression or anxiety, are eliminated.[16] It also causes cognitive impairments, especially disruptions in attention, verbal memory, and new learning even after controlling for attention problems and IQ.[17] Thus it must be addressed directly, via evidence-based treatments such as cognitive processing therapy, individual and group CBT, individual eye-movement desensitization and reprocessing (EMDR) or pharmacotherapy.[18]

Depression, substance abuse, and adjustment disorder are also possible diagnoses for someone with Marcus's presentation, and we'd routinely be alert for these in all college students. Less common student problems, such as traumatic brain injury, are more frequent among veterans. There's growing recognition that even a single exposure to an explosion, such as from the improvised explosive devices common in the recent wars, can lead to microscopic changes in the brain that translate into difficulties with learning and memory, as well as other psychological symptoms.[19] This is similar to the chronic traumatic encephalopathy suffered by some athletes who have experienced repeated concussions, but in the case of veterans, a blast rather than a head blow may be to blame, and neither veteran nor physician may correctly identify the problem without being aware of this link. Traumatic brain injuries can cause personality changes and irritability as well as interfere with a student veteran's ability to succeed not only in the classroom but in social settings as well. And a student who has PTSD *and* a traumatic brain injury faces extra challenges.

Effective work with Marcus requires us to understand both military culture and campus culture as well as some of the unique challenges that arise when a student makes this transition. Programs are springing up to help educate mental health professionals about these variables, including the JED Foundation's online course, "Understanding and Supporting the Emotional Health of Student Veterans." This overview of common problems and treatment approaches in working with this group of students is a great starting point. The U.S. Department of Veterans Affairs has also developed online resources for student veterans and for the campus health professionals who work with them. These include descriptions of military culture and battlefield skills, accounts of common adjustment issues that arise in the transition to college, and CME-certified online trainings focused on "the silent wounds of war."

Female student veterans may face additional challenges. Many women experienced gender discrimination while deployed, both from within the male-dominated military and from people in the countries in which they served. Some experienced sexual or physical trauma in addition to the trauma of combat. We must remain sensitive to these issues and refer as appropriate for additional services.

Most university campuses have a Veterans Services Office which helps student veterans negotiate financial and administrative issues related to their student status, but the level of services differs significantly from one institution to another.[20] Still, it's helpful to be aware of these services and to refer students to them as appropriate. Some find the transition from a highly regimented life with a clear hierarchy to the freedom of college life daunting, and may need help with learning to structure their time.

Another important issue in working with student veterans is to help them consider whether they may qualify for disability accommodations. Universities follow the Americans with Disabilities Act guidelines to determine eligibility for accommodations, but the Department of Veterans Affairs uses its own guidelines. Thus, a student may have applied for and been denied VA benefits for a disability but may still qualify for academic accommodations on campus based on ADA guidelines.

As the numbers of nontraditional students on campus increase, these students might also benefit from campus-wide interventions, including outreach and preventive health workshops that specifically address their needs. Creating student veteran groups might help alleviate the sense of isolation that returning veterans feel. The University of Arizona created SERV (Supportive Education for Returning Veterans), a three-course program that includes resilience skills and a "crash course in how to succeed" in college and helps students understand their own learning styles.[21] Their student veteran retention rates are 95%. Mental health professionals can collaborate with other campus organizations and offices to tailor support groups or other sorts of gatherings to meet the unique needs of these and other nontraditional students. As psychiatrists we can also provide psychoeducation and consultation to faculty members about the sorts of cognitive challenges that students with PTSD or traumatic brain injuries may face, as well as other information about the effectiveness of various teaching styles on older or otherwise nontraditional students.

Students with Disabilities

Esther, a 19-year-old sophomore from New York, presents to her first appointment walking with the assistance of two crutches, sweating and short of breath after having climbed several flights to the counseling center offices.

She insists it's not a problem for her to get to the office but starts to cry as soon as the door is shut. She has felt increasingly down the last three weeks, tired, and not wanting to engage in social activities. She has cerebral palsy, "but I've lived with that my whole life and have gotten good at breaking stereotypes." She and her family had been elated at how well she'd adapted to college life in her freshman year, but now, after being accepted to her first choice sorority, she feels increasingly isolated because she can't participate in many of the sorority's social events. An incident after a party this weekend left her particularly upset. She'd gotten drunk and woken up in bed with a young man she'd really liked. But he asked her to leave, and since then has acted like he barely knows her.

In the last twenty years, the number of students with disabilities on the college campus has doubled.[22] Disabilities can be physically apparent to others, as in Esther's case, or invisible. Because they can affect a student's life in such a variety of ways, from impairments in physical mobility to special senses (hearing or vision impairments) to learning disabilities to psychiatric ones, discussing them as a group omits much. But in general for psychiatrists and others working with students with mental health concerns, a general sensitivity to this subgroup of nontraditional students and attention to some of the common challenges they may face is important.

Students with disabilities must navigate all the normal developmental challenges of students without, but sometimes they also have to cope with additional developmental, medical, and logistical challenges that can affect their emotional well-being. In the transition from high school to college, they often must shift from a passive reliance on many others who advocate for and take care of their needs—parents, school systems, personalized Individualized Education Plans—to an active role in managing their disability.[23] This means contacting the appropriate offices at their institutions, self-identifying as having a disability, and providing necessary documentation. It often means learning to advocate for their own needs in specific situations. At a developmental stage when independence from family and fitting into peer groups is important, it can be especially hard to have a condition that requires some dependence on others, and that makes a student stand out in what they may perceive as a negative way.

Youth with disabilities may have been especially protected by their parents during high school, limiting their autonomy and making the transition to the freedom of college life particularly abrupt and complex. They may be at a younger social developmental stage than their chronological age, and it's important to remember this in our work with them. They may engage in riskier behavior, like adolescents. Until recently, there were almost no data on determinants of health in college students with disabilities. The 2008 American College Health Association–National College Health Assessment II (ACHA-NCHA II) allowed students to identify their disability as research participants, and one study of over 60,000 American college students from more than 100 institutions specifically compared the substance use and sexual risk behaviors of students with disabilities to those of students without.[24] This study found that 12.5% of the sample reported having one disability, and 4.6% reported two or more disabilities. Compared to students without disabilities, those with disabilities were more likely to engage in substance use risk behaviors (including heavy drinking, drinking and driving, and diagnosis of addiction), and those with two or more disabilities had a higher odds ratio than those with a single disability. A similar trend emerged for sexually risky behaviors: students with disabilities reported more sexual partners, lower rates of condom use with all types of sex, and higher rates of unintentional pregnancy. The authors of the study suggest that, contrary to stereotypes suggesting that people with disabilities are asexual or less sexually active or desirable, this group is actually quite sexually active and may be especially vulnerable to health risks. Because the two most common disabilities in this group were ADHD and "psychiatric condition," this information is perhaps less surprising to us as psychiatrists, but the top third condition was "chronic illness," and those with mobility or other disabling conditions were also represented.

Interestingly, in this study, students with disabilities were also more likely to be from an ethnic minority group than students without disabilities, to identify as biracial or multiracial, and to identify as gay or bisexual. This suggests that people with disabilities may be part of two or more marginalized groups on campus, leading to greater potential problems with loneliness and isolation.

In Esther's case, it's important to do a thorough psychiatric assessment, including substance use and sexual risk behaviors, given her presenting concern, and then to also help her examine how she's integrating living with a disability into her developing sense of herself as an emerging adult. Her disability may be completely irrelevant to her experience of feeling rejected by the young man, whose behavior may have been identical with any other woman. Or, he may in fact have treated her badly because of her difference. Either way allowing her to explore these concerns is important.

We should also pay attention to the physical space of our offices and accommodate students who have difficulty getting up stairs. Ideally all our offices would be accessible, but in many older university buildings, we must navigate stairs and tight corners that don't accommodate wheelchairs. Until buildings can be retrofitted, an alternative space in which to meet students who might have difficulty getting to a non-accessible office is helpful. In my experience, even students like Esther, who insist they can make it up the stairs, are grateful for alternative arrangements that don't require them to make that extra effort. And it's always helpful to check in with students regarding their accommodations and explore whether these are in fact working for them. Sometimes they need support in returning to the Office for Students with Disabilities to advocate further for their needs, which may change with the changing demands of university life.

CHAPTER 20

Models of Treatment

Carrie, a 21-year old Southeast-Asian (Indian) American junior, comes in complaining of depressive symptoms and declining academic performance. She begins sheepishly with "I did something stupid. I stopped my medicine." She was seen for similar complaints a year ago and treated with an antidepressant, which helped; however, she'd discontinued the medicine after two months because she'd felt better, and when summer began, she did not follow through with the therapy that had been recommended. Many of her depressive symptoms are triggered by complex conflicts within her family, from whom she was mostly apart over the summer. In the fall she was abroad. There were times when she felt depressed, and she drank more heavily while abroad, but overall she felt stable. Lately she's getting drawn into her parents' ongoing discord as well as severe family financial problems. The record reveals that she attended two sessions of therapy at the counseling center the previous year and two medication management visits and that she was improving but then stopped coming to either therapy or medication management and was lost to follow-up.

Many of the models of psychiatric treatment in which most of us psychiatrists were trained meet challenges in working with college students. It's not uncommon for students to discontinue their medication earlier than recommended, or to avoid or prematurely terminate therapy. Often it's not out of resistance or a desire to be noncompliant. Shifting our focus from a pathology-based model to a developmental framework, we can better understand that emerging adults are just beginning to learn to take responsibility for their own health and wellness. They may equate mental health treatment with being mentally ill, and thus, at the first signs of feeling better, they flee treatment in the hope that discarding it also discards the possibility that something is wrong. They may attribute feeling better to a misdiagnosis in the first place and question the need for ongoing care. Or something as simple as the academic year calendar, with its multiple hiatuses—vacations, breaks, and study abroad—may disrupt their resolve to engage in ongoing treatment.

A core developmental task of emerging adulthood is managing the change from "dependency on one's parents and other older adults to independence,"[1] and this comes in conflict with traditional models of mental health care, including long-term but even briefer forms of regular psychotherapy and ongoing medication management. These can seem to encourage dependence. Even though today's generation of students is more connected with their parents, keeping in closer touch and relying on them for advice, their trajectory through college still involves developing healthy autonomy, and this may play out in a student's attitudes toward treatment.

The fact is that many students do well even without ongoing long-term treatment. Those dealing with recurrent conditions, such as major depression or an anxiety disorder, will find themselves needing continued treatment. It's important for the psychiatrist they see not to shame them for their treatment interruption and to remain flexible regarding the modes of treatment that will fit students' needs. Psychologist Richard Eichler, who is director of Columbia's counseling center, also recommends meeting many students' abrupt cessation of counseling with an invitation to return when and if the student likes, noting that allowing them to use counseling intermittently actually supports their efforts at individuation.[2] He suggests that college students are better able to make forays into the wider world with the knowledge of a secure base to which they can return in a crisis; most of us working in university settings have experienced this firsthand.

As psychiatrists recommending a medical treatment, though, we must walk a fine line between understanding the developmental perspective and informing students about the recommended duration of medication treatment and risks of early discontinuation. At the same time, we must normalize their experiences with premature discontinuation as these arise. A student presenting with Carrie's concerns, who may have had a depressive disorder with good response to an antidepressant, is likely to respond again, and we can easily resume medication. In my experience, some students meet full criteria for a mood or anxiety disorder while on campus, but do seem to do much better, even without treatment, at other times in other settings. Whether this implies that the original diagnosis was incorrect, or that emerging adults in college settings may have somewhat different symptom presentations or even treatment needs than the adults on whom diagnostic criteria were normed, is unclear, but more research on college student populations would be helpful in addressing these patterns and especially in understanding how and when offering medication treatment might be most appropriate.

Although most college counseling centers have to limit treatment in order to match resources to student needs, psychiatrists treating students solely with medication management may be able to work with students over a longer period. Especially once a student is stabilized, their visits can be more distantly spaced. It's easy to get swept up in the mind frame of referring out all students who may need treatment for longer than a specified time, but most students taking medicine will need more than just a few months of treatment, and the psychiatrist who first saw them may be the most appropriate person to provide that treatment. If we consider that a student with recurrent major depression who has responded to an SSRI may need to see the psychiatrist only three times in an academic year, for 30-minute sessions, then ongoing treatment with the same provider may tax the system less than referring the student out, only to have him drop out of treatment and return later in crisis. Some stabilized students can be referred out to primary care providers for medication refills, but the contact with a psychiatrist can also provide brief psychotherapy "booster shots," or at the least an opportunity to fine-tune the treatment and re-evaluate student concerns. It also helps model for students the importance of a consistent relationship. One study has shown that college students receiving antidepressant medication from a psychiatrist are significantly more likely to receive "minimally adequate" treatment than those seeing a primary care provider.[3] One hopes that we're all raising the bar higher than minimally adequate, but at least this threshold seems more likely with consistent psychiatric treatment.

When a student like Carrie returns, expressing some shame at her previous nonadherence to treatment, it may be a logical moment to refer her out for ongoing care, but this might reinforce her sense that she has done something wrong and make it less likely that she will actually follow through with a referral. Another option is to provide "bridge" care, planning with the student from the outset to meet for a limited number of sessions, until she's again feeling better, and then to refer out with the hope that the initial good experience with developing a trusting relationship, and the emphasis on education within the bridging work, will encourage the student to seek a similar relationship with a recommended private practice physician.

Episodic or intermittent treatment thus becomes the norm in work with the college student population. As psychotherapy in general in the United States has moved toward briefer models, more therapists (and patients) expect therapy to be time limited. A number of studies have supported the efficacy of brief therapy in working with emerging adults. There's less evidence on the efficacy of other models of intermittent treatment. For example, many students prefer not to meet weekly, and ask for every other week or even monthly sessions. This helps centers manage resources, and therapists are more willing these days to accommodate these requests or even to suggest regular but infrequent meetings. Again, more research on outcomes would greatly help determine whether these are equally good as, or perhaps better or worse than, more traditional weekly patterns of care.

Group Treatments

College students are used to group situations. Much of their social lives, their living arrangements, and their academic activities happen in groups. Yet they can be reluctant when referred to group treatments for emotional problems. Some of this may be due to campus culture, which emphasizes competence and success and creates fear of admitting vulnerability. Many clinicians, too, shy away from considering group as a first-line treatment modality. This is unfortunate, since the evidence suggests that groups are actually an extremely effective way for students to experience improvement in many of the concerns that bring them to counseling.

Groups have shown efficacy with adjustment and developmental concerns in college students as well as with more significant psychopathology, and some suggest group psychotherapy is the treatment of choice for concerns around autonomy, intimacy, and self-esteem.[4] Furthermore, the more general factors in any group therapy, including socialization, interpersonal skills, and universality, may be especially therapeutic for college students, perhaps more so than specific theoretical orientations. In one randomized controlled study comparing group CBT for social anxiety with a more general group therapy approach, both led to significant improvement among college students, and the approach that paid more attention to group processes actually had fewer drop-outs.[5] Groups with specific theoretical orientations, such as dialectical behavior therapy (DBT), can be extremely helpful for certain problems, including eating disorders, borderline personality symptoms (such as self-harm or suicidal thinking), or other difficulties with emotional regulation.

Group treatments also have the advantage of being able to draw in students from the nonclinical population, and as such they can begin to shift campus culture toward healthier norms. This can enhance resilience in the population in general and perhaps prevent the onset of more serious problems in susceptible students. For example, at Duke University psychologist Gary Glass and colleagues have developed a broad palette of "developmental programming," which includes workshops, classes, and even groups that combine emotional and physical exercise modalities.

We've long had mindfulness meditation groups led by psychiatrist Holly Rogers, to which clinicians can refer their clients but to which students who have never used the counseling center can also self-refer. These have grown in popularity and are now the focus of research. There's growing evidence that mindfulness practice has significant benefits to brain-body health. These include quantifiable benefits such as increased prefrontal cortical activity and reduced amygdala activation during an affect-labeling task in undergraduates disposed to mindfulness, and increased salivary antibodies and decreased cortisol in college students exposed to stress after a mindfulness-based intervention.[6] Good data suggest that mindfulness meditation decreases physiological stress responses and as such can lower anxiety and depression. We now have an additional group combining yoga with mindfulness.

Other recent programs have included a "worrying well" group, which teaches CBT and other techniques to combat anxiety and excessive worry; a "stress for success" workshop; programs for first-generation college students; and groups focused on a particular aspect of a student's identity, such as international status, gender, or ethnicity. Making these groups normative and more visible within the college community also decreases the stigma associated with visiting the counseling center. In addition to providing much needed services, these groups can serve as a conduit for students who are more at risk for significant illness, encouraging them to consider individual evaluations when appropriate. Groups also combat isolation and social hopelessness, which are risk factors for suicide in college students.

Combining good group therapy with medication management may be one very effective model of care for college students with psychiatric concerns. It makes intuitive sense but has not been systematically studied. In these cases, the psychiatrist remains the student's primary caregiver and should check in periodically with group leaders to find out how their shared patient is faring. For a student like Carrie, , especially if she is reluctant to engage in individual therapy, a mindfulness group or an interpersonal group might be extremely helpful.

Integrated Treatment, Split Treatment, and Referral

Given the growing complexity of students' mental health needs and the fact that one student may be receiving multiple types of treatment, integrated care remains important but challenging. Different centers have varying practices regarding combined treatment. Some counseling centers choose not to pre-scribe medications for students who are not also in therapy, in keeping with a developmental perspective regarding all student emotional concerns. As our understanding of mood and anxiety disorders has grown, though, this seems an unreasonably rigid standard to apply across the board. Although almost everyone could likely benefit from therapy—and this is particularly true of students with depression and anxiety—student preference and clinical indica-tion are better guides for when to pair therapy with medication management. In many cases it is entirely within the standard of care to treat a student just with medicine, or just with therapy. If resources permit direct referral to a psy-chiatrist for students who request this, or for students being referred in from other providers, such as student health, for example, in many cases this is very appropriate.

When students are treated with both medicine and therapy, however, it's im-portant for the therapist and psychiatrist to communicate and coordinate care. This is much more easily accomplished when both are working within the same counseling center. Sometimes a weekly interdisciplinary team meeting is the perfect place to touch base about shared patients. At other times this is accom-plished via a brief consultation, in person or over the phone. It's much harder to treat collaboratively if one part of the treatment is taking place within the counseling center, and another in the community. Given the constraints on resources, some centers choose not to "split" treatment: that is, if a student is referred out for ongoing therapy, then medication management is also referred out. Likewise, if a student has an established relationship with a community therapist, then she may be referred to a community psychiatrist for medication needs.

If a student taking medicine is not in individual therapy, the psychiatrist needs to play more of a coordinating role in recommending other services. Group therapy, career counseling, or referral to a nutritionist may all be important parts of the treatment, and the more the psychiatrist collaborates with the other providers involved, the better the care will be.

Some student concerns are best treated in a more intensive, open-ended model than the counseling center can provide. Most chronic conditions, including psychotic disorders, many cases of bipolar disorder, problems related to significant trauma, many eating disorders, and addictions are most effectively treated by a specialized clinician who does not have the length-of-treatment limitations of campus providers. The decision to refer out should not be based just on diagnosis, however. It should take into account the individual student's current state and the anticipated ongoing clinical needs. For example, a student with bipolar disorder who is stable on medications and has had a course of treatment, who presents with distress over a relationship break-up and wants to do brief therapy around the break-up before graduating in a few months, might benefit from working with a psychology intern within the counseling center, while another student, newly diagnosed with bipolar disorder and struggling with excessive drug use, poor impulse control, and grief over the diagnosis, would gain more from a stable ongoing relationship with a provider who will be available to her more frequently and for the duration of the next four years of her graduate studies.

Even when it's clear that referral out is the optimal disposition, however, bridging to the referral by providing a few weeks of stabilizing treatment can be invaluable. It's usually not a good idea to refer a student out in the midst of a crisis. Timing of the referral is important and challenging: we don't want to encourage too much attachment in a student who will need more extensive services, but we don't want to create a sense of rejection or abandonment in a student in the midst of crisis. Framing the treatment as bridging treatment, and explicitly telling the student that we will work together with them to find a good treatment match, is helpful.

Treatment Hiatuses

Students go home for breaks and vacations and occasionally are gone for entire semesters or years of study abroad. If they're taking medication, planning for these interruptions in treatment is important. Some students have a psychiatrist or primary care doctor at home who takes over their care over breaks. Again, communication between providers is critical to continuity of care. When a student travels and wants to continue treatment, the precise nature of the plan depends on clinical judgment and the student's status when last evaluated on campus. The student who comes to the counseling center for the first time with a mood or anxiety disorder, just weeks before leaving for six months abroad, is probably not best served by a prescription that will last the entirety of that time away. In these cases, whenever possible, it makes sense to start the student on medicine, have a follow-up visit or at minimum phone check-in to assess tolerability, and then refer the student to a provider in the country to which he is traveling. But students who are known to the psychiatrist because of a well-established treatment relationship, and who are stable at the time they go abroad, often do well if they're given enough medication to last them while they're away, with a plan to return for re-evaluation when they get back.

Medical leave is a special kind of treatment hiatus. When a student goes on medical leave for a psychological or psychiatric reason, the psychiatrist can play a critical role in setting up clear expectations for care while the student is away. Too often students leave campus and don't follow treatment recommendations, only to flail once again upon their return to campus. Whenever possible, it's helpful to collaborate with deans or other administrative staff to clearly delineate for the student expectations for treatment, emphasizing that the successful completion of these might affect the student's odds of being re-admitted to the university community. Some universities are putting uniform policies in place that specify expectations for treatment when students take a medical leave. Far from being punitive—though emerging adults might initially view them this way—these policies protect students by ensuring that they make good use of their time away, and that they return to campus healthier than they were when they left, and thus better able to meet the challenges of college life.

CHAPTER 21

Treatment Challenges in the University Population

Treating university students is fun and professionally rewarding work. They're bright, motivated, and interesting, and the very issue that's most challenging in their care—distinguishing normal developmental phases from more significant emerging psychopathology—is also what keeps the work intriguing and fulfilling. That particular complexity has been addressed throughout the other chapters of this book. Some of these other challenges, briefly summarized below, are also discussed as relevant in other sections.

Prescribing Issues

The two main obstacles that arise in treating students with psychotropic medicine are related to one another. The first is that many whom we think would benefit are reluctant to take medication. The second, which may partly explain their reluctance, is that these young adults seem to have a slightly different side effect profile than older adults or are more aware and less tolerant of side effects.

Reluctance to Take Medicine

College students resist taking antidepressant, mood-stabilizing, or antipsychotic medicines for many reasons. Sometimes resistance is a based on cultural beliefs: the prevailing viewpoint in their country or community of origin might be that depression or anxiety are not illnesses and therefore can't be improved by medicine. Sometimes they've seen a friend or family member react badly to a medication. Some equate needing the medicine with being defective or mentally ill, and therefore they believe that getting well "on their own" will demonstrate that they never needed medicine and thus were never ill. Anxious students will have read up on every possible side effect and every report of a bad reaction, and this fuels their fear. Sometimes student reluctance is an appropriate response for their developmental stage. As they're trying to become autonomous, competent adults, the idea of "needing" a medication for longer than a week or two conjures up fears of dependence or incapacitation.

For some students the cost of medicine is prohibitive. Even with insurance, some copays may be above the student's budget, and if he doesn't want to reveal to his family that he's taking medicine, this becomes an obstacle. Sometimes, the student has heard that medication is being "overprescribed" and wants to ensure that's not the case for him.

Students tend to be up-to-date on the latest articles in circulation, and when these challenge the efficacy of medicine for depression, for example, they pay attention. When a large meta-analysis of antidepressants suggested that drugs were not significantly better than placebo for mild to moderate depression,[1] for example, more students balked at the option of medication treatment. In cases of mild to moderate depression, there's enough evidence to suggest that it's reasonable to try exercise, therapy, or other stress-reducing treatments first, including mindfulness meditation or yoga.[2] But often the students who come to a psychiatrist have already tried these options without success. In those cases, an in-depth discussion of the article that worried them, explaining the limitations of the study (in the case cited above, short duration, small number of studies, one-drug trials, etc.) can alleviate the student's concerns and allow them to get relief.

It's important to take the time to understand exactly what an individual student's concerns are when she refuses medicine. Then, taking a collaborative stance, we can provide accurate information and our own recommendation, while making it clear to the student that ultimately the decision is theirs. It's always good practice to review alternative treatments and to avoid an authoritarian stance or power struggles over the exact treatment. Obviously this applies only when the students' cognitive abilities are intact and they have good insight and judgment. If a student is psychotic or manic, or there are other indications that not treating would lead to imminent danger, then we have to consider involuntary hospitalization and involuntary treatment. Fortunately, this last scenario is quite rare in college mental health work (but for a more in-depth discussion of what to do when it does occur, refer to chapter 17).

Occasionally, the opposite problem occurs—a student comes in requesting or demanding a medicine that is not, in our opinion, clinically indicated. A student may have tried his roommate's stimulant and decided he has ADHD (see chapter 13), or may have had a course of treatment for depression earlier and now requests medicine at the first sign of dysphoria. Students may request sleeping medicine or benzodiazepines after trying these from friends or family members, or in response to direct-to-consumer advertising. Their specific request does not automatically preclude that the treatment may in fact be appropriate for their problem, but we can't bypass the step of a full evaluation to determine whether this is the case.

Medication Side Effects

Students are sensitive to any side effects that might compromise their ability to study or to socialize. There are almost no data on differential side effect profiles among college students compared to other populations, but many clinicians with experience working with this population think there may be differences. In a small open-label pilot study that colleagues and I conducted at Duke University's Counseling and Psychological Services (CAPS), of students treated with the most commonly prescribed antidepressants, those older than 25 reported more drowsiness, impaired sleep, and unsteadiness than students aged 18 to 24, although 20% of even the younger group complained of drowsiness.[3] Non-Caucasian students seemed more sensitive to dizziness (33% versus 10%), and Caucasian students seemed more sensitive to sexual side effects (22% compared with 0%). Of course, that latter number may have more to do with lack of reporting side effects, perhaps out of a cultural reticence to discuss sexuality or simply because the sample size was too small to capture the side effect. In my clinical experience non-Caucasian students do report sexual side effects at similar rates to Caucasian students when all are routinely asked the same questions. Anecdotally, drowsiness and sexual side effects limit the usefulness of SSRIs among students a bit more frequently than is reported in the literature for the general population.

Students seem to disproportionately fear weight gain from antidepressants, perhaps because of the high rate of eating and body image concerns among this population. Some students do gain weight, but again, good data on the exact numbers, especially by specific medicine, are lacking. In my clinical experience weight gain is not common with the SSRIs, but in the rare instances when it occurs, it can be significant. The rule of thumb prescribing for students is to start at very low doses and slowly titrate upward to the therapeutic range. Discussing potential side effects first, and clarifying that side effects precede beneficial effects and usually are short lived, makes it much more likely that students will continue a medicine long enough to at least assess efficacy.

Other Prescribing Challenges

It's not uncommon for college students to self-treat their emotional concerns with herbal medication. Studies suggest that about a quarter to half of college students use herbal remedies, a higher rate than in the general population; that over a third use these to treat a mood or emotional problem, and that only a quarter disclosed this use to their healthcare providers.[4] Furthermore, there's significant overlap between the students who take an herbal preparation and those who also take a prescription medication. Although many herbal treatments have relatively few side effects on their own, in combination with other medicine, they can cause or exacerbate side effects. St. John's wort in particular can have additive effects with SSRIs. It's important therefore to specifically ask about alternative or complementary medicines, and even to name one or two since some students consider them "herbs" and not drugs.

Another prescribing challenge is that college life is full of interruptions: breaks, vacations, and time abroad (see chapter 20 for more on treatment hiatuses). This raises the question of how ethically and practically sound it is to continue to provide treatment for someone whom we can't assess for an extended period. Decisions whether to continue treatment by providing multiple refills must be made on a case-by-case basis, using sound clinical judgment. Students who are stable and have a long record of good self-care and keeping appointments are likely best served by continued treatment over breaks, with the understanding that they contact us if anything changes and that they may then need referral to a local physician. In those cases it's good practice to discuss contingent and emergency plans should a crisis arise. Some students are not stable enough to be sent home with multiple refills, or have not been in treatment long enough to develop a good treatment alliance or for the psychiatrist to feel confident in accurately assessing their needs. These students will need referral to a psychiatrist near their home. It's important to be very clear about who is treating the student when, and to get releases to communicate with the outside providers. Practicing and documenting good continuity of care is essential in order for students to maintain the treatment gains they make.

More complex is when a student travels abroad for a semester or other extended period of time. Again, decisions can be made case by case. If the student is well-known to the psychiatrist, has been stable and treatment adherent, and needs continued medication management, it might be reasonable to provide a four- or five-month supply of an antidepressant. But some countries have different laws governing which medicines can be legally brought in, even with a prescription and for personal use. For example, Japan has very restrictive laws, limiting the prescription medication allowance to a one-month supply and forbidding certain classes of medication entirely, including prescription and over-the-counter stimulants. It's best to ask students to research, via their destination country's embassy, policies around medication. Sometimes there's a process of advance application and paperwork for permission to bring in more than a month's worth of medicine, as in Japan. The option of getting refills from a physician abroad might be less complicated, however, and have the added advantage of ongoing follow-up care for the student. Sometimes students need help navigating ways to find psychiatrists or therapists abroad, and often this can be coordinated through the university's office of study abroad.

Occasionally a student is doing well taking a medication that is not available in identical form in the country to which she'll be traveling. In those cases, she'll need to consult with a physician as soon as possible upon arrival abroad. If it is a clinically appropriate time to consider treatment discontinuation, it's important to do this far enough in advance of their departure date that the transitions of going abroad don't confound the diagnostic picture.

Individual Student Needs versus University Community Needs

High-profile tragedies, such as the Virginia Tech massacre in 2007 and the cluster of suicides at Cornell in 2009–2010, lead to reappraisals of the systems in place for taking care of the most significantly disturbed students. But legal and ethical challenges make it difficult to uniformly address all the complex situations that arise on campus. Behavioral intervention teams are a good starting point. These now meet regularly at many universities and systematically review "students of concern," identified via reports from faculty, medical personnel, or other students. But there are ongoing tensions between individual student rights, such as the right to privacy, confidentiality, and even refusal of treatment, and the university community's need to maintain order, safety, and effective functioning. Furthermore, although most university students are legal adults, the closer ties of the current generation of students to their families means that parents often have higher expectations that they be kept in the loop by universities whenever situations of concern arise with their children.

But the notion of confidentiality is an essential one in mental health treatment, key not only to students' willingness to seek help and share personal and potentially embarrassing or even incriminating information, but also legally protected under state and federal laws, and under HIPAA and FERPA (the Family Educational Rights and Privacy Act). HIPAA does not always apply to college counseling centers, but it does in some instances. With the widespread implementation of electronic medical records, and the increasing use of these systems at counseling centers too, it's likely that more and more psychiatrists treating college students will be operating under HIPAA and not just FERPA. It also makes good clinical sense for psychiatrists to be able to communicate about psychiatric treatment, especially medication management, with other physicians and health care providers treating a student. And because university personnel outside the health care setting are governed not by HIPAA but by FERPA, sometimes they can disclose information in the best interest of the student that could not be disclosed by a physician under HIPAA.

Experts on how the legal framework applies to college student issues recommend that schools continue to uphold confidentiality in compliance with the state or federal law with the strictest requirements.[5] However, they also remind us that appropriate allowances for disclosure *do* exist, and that often college mental health providers, faculty, and administrators misinterpret or don't know the details of privacy laws or FERPA, leading to unnecessary withholding of information that could potentially help in a difficult situation.

For example, FERPA, which governs what university personnel may share about a student's educational record, does *not* protect personal knowledge that a university member may have about a student's behavior from being shared without the student's consent.[6] This means that professors who are concerned about a student's repeated absences from class, for example, or RAs who observe a student repeatedly purging in the bathroom, or deans who are contacted because a student is in the emergency room with an alcohol-related injury, can in fact share that information without the student's consent. This has to be done judiciously, in the interest of helping the student, and preferably with consent. But it always makes sense for university personnel who are worried about a student's behavior to consult at the very least with counseling center staff, without fearing they're violating privacy rules.

Conversely, when a psychiatrist has a release to speak with faculty or other university personnel about a student's worrisome mental health problems, the psychiatrist can remind the other person that under FERPA, *they* can notify the student's parents if that disclosure is likely to help the student, even if the psychiatrist can't, as long as the disclosure falls under one of the many allowances under FERPA.

Todd, a 19-year-old Caucasian sophomore, comes in for an emergency evaluation at the insistence of his dean, who got him to sign a consent for two-way release of information with the psychiatrist. Several professors are concerned that he has been missing classes and even exams, and he is at risk of academic dismissal. Todd describes a two-month period of increasingly sad and then apathetic mood, inability to concentrate, anhedonia, and hopelessness. Much of this started after failure to be admitted to any of the fraternities he rushed. His main coping strategy has been to increase his drinking, alone in his room. He does not have a roommate but admits that two friends have expressed worry about his drinking. He dismisses this, insisting the alcohol is not a problem. He denies suicidal or homicidal thoughts. He is unshaven, slightly malodorous, and wears rumpled clothing. He has not been showering or eating regularly and has "maybe" lost some weight.

Todd agrees to treatment. He believes he can "pull it together" and refuses to consider a medical leave. He does not want his parents contacted, stating that he does not want to worry them—his father was recently laid off, and his mother has been in poor health. However, he does not keep follow-up appointments for therapy or medication management. He does not respond to phone calls or other attempts by counseling center staff to reach him.

Psychiatrists can always break confidentiality in emergency situations, but more complex are the cases where imminent risk is not clear yet failure to act will in all probability lead to deterioration and possibly even harm. Todd is clearly either depressed or suffering from a substance-induced mood disorder. His isolation and withdrawal from school are very concerning. But the most likely outcome at this moment is academic dismissal, not necessarily imminent medical harm. Is this sufficient grounds for violating confidentiality? Because he gave consent for communication with the dean, this would be a good first step for the psychiatrist after other attempts at reaching the student have failed.

Todd's dean is similarly frustrated with the difficulty of reaching the student but reports that the RA checked in with Todd, brought him pizza, and said Todd was still denying any intent to harm himself. However, there were several empty vodka bottles in the dorm room. The dean and psychiatrist agree that a medical leave is appropriate and would be more beneficial for the student than academic dismissal, since it might compel him to get treatment and allow him to more easily return to school once he is ready. They confer about breaking confidentiality and contacting Todd's family.

Under FERPA, multiple provisions allow for disclosure in a case like this. For example, this dean could contact the family because the student is under 21 and violating university alcohol policies, or because this situation constitutes a health emergency.[7] In the wake of Virginia Tech, FERPA guidelines were somewhat loosened to remove the "strictly construed" provision of what constitutes a medical emergency. This underscores recognition that colleges have "greater flexibility and deference to bring appropriate resources to bear on a circumstance that threatens the health or safety of individuals."[8] And considering the generational attitudes of today's parents, who expect universities to protect and care for their children much more comprehensively than in the past, as well as the attitudes of the students themselves, who have been raised in a much more protected and structured environment than previous generations, university faculty often have more discretion to disclose information than they believe they do.

Sometimes the student's objection to disclosure may be based on their developmentally appropriate wish to maintain independence. Occasionally it's based on an illogical wish to protect their parents from the difficult realities of the student's situation, illogical because clearly sooner or later the parents will find out. In Todd's case, it's better to notify them earlier, in the interest of enlisting their help in getting Todd into treatment. No one can force a student to take a medical leave, but many universities do have mandatory leave policies in place. For example, at Stanford, if a student "is unable or unwilling to carry out substantial self-care obligations or to participate meaningfully in educational activities," he can be compelled to take a Dean's Leave of Absence.[9] In cases where the student's judgment may be impairing his ability to weigh benefits versus costs of taking a leave, having family step in can be a reasonable and often helpful step.

It's important for psychiatrists to continually balance the clinical needs of the student against the wishes and needs of family and university. Because there has been litigation where colleges were found liable for student suicide based on the notion of a "special relationship" between a university and its students, some universities have created policies that force students to take a medical leave if they express suicidal thoughts or in other ways engage in potentially endangering behavior.[10] For example, some schools have barred students from their dorm or from campus after treatment for a suicide attempt, or compelled students with a history of suicidal thoughts and depression to take a medical leave even when the student and her psychiatrist felt she was improving enough that she could safely continue in school. Although these cases are likely complex, and the schools may have had good reason to act as they did, legal experts caution against acting in a way that seems designed to protect the university from legal liability, rather than to maximally support the student. Stigma is already such a barrier to students' seeking mental health treatment; if they were to fear losing their student status as a result of reporting depressive or suicidal thoughts, how many more might avoid treatment?

Suicide Prevention

The rate of suicide among youth ages 15 to 24 has increased in the last 50 years, and suicide is the second leading cause of death for students on college campuses, claiming more than 1,000 lives each year.[11] Contrary to earlier reports, however, college actually seems to have a protective effect on emerging adults. A well-regarded study by Morton Silverman and colleagues of completed suicides at 12 midwestern colleges found that students died by suicide at a rate of about half that of age-matched nonstudent young adults.[12] They attributed this to a number of factors, including the availability of free or low-cost health care services, limited access to firearms, a supportive community, and a sense of purpose among students. The student suicide rate has been estimated at between 6.5 and 7.5/100,000 per year over the last two decades.

So although it doesn't seem like the rate is actually *increasing* among college students, it remains stubbornly stable, and each potentially preventable death is tragic. As attitudes change, with parents and others expecting more and more of colleges in terms of protecting their children, suicide prevention has received increased attention. Most college students who commit suicide are not current or former patients of the counseling center; in fact, evidence suggests that counseling center treatment greatly reduces the risk of suicide.[13] The problem is identifying at-risk students and encouraging them to engage in treatment, or in other activities that might reduce risk. In a screening project at Emory sponsored by the American Foundation for Suicide Prevention, 11% of students reported suicidal ideation in the past month, yet 84% of these students were not receiving any psychiatric treatment at the time, despite a high incidence of depression among this group.[14]

Certain groups of students—older students, veterans, those who identify as LGBT, and some minority groups, such as American Indians—are at greater risk. Students who enter college with a history of mental health problems are also more at risk. Depression, hopelessness, and loneliness have all been identified as potent factors in suicidal ideation, with some studies finding the strongest association for depression. Recent negative life events, previous attempts, alcohol, substance abuse, and insomnia all increase risk. As is the case for other age groups, men commit suicide more frequently than women. Social hopelessness is a particularly important variable in this age group: students remain hopeful about their abilities and academics, for example, but feel socially isolated and socially incompetent, and this increases their risk of self-harm. Women have an increased risk of suicide in the 30 days after an attempted nonconsensual sexual penetration, and with high levels of alcohol, while for men a physical or sexual assault in the past year increases risk.[15]

A lot of the research on suicide prevention focuses on community-wide efforts that try to identify at-risk individuals and target the campus climate to reduce factors that might lead to or exacerbate depression among students. Outreach programming that focuses not only on educational programs but also on experiential programs such as stress reduction workshops and relationship improvement groups has the potential to benefit many students, including those who might be at risk of suicide. Psychiatrists can be involved in these programs, to increase their own visibility, making themselves more "real" and less threatening to students, and to provide a bio-psycho-social perspective.

But it's clear that suicide prevention on campus isn't the province of just the mental health practitioners. Research shows that educating many campus constituencies—from faculty and administrators to students and families, as much as possible—to recognize signs of depression, hopelessness, and possible suicidal thinking can strengthen the safety net for students. The JED Foundation stresses that the behavioral intervention teams that many universities formed in response to campus violence have an important role in monitoring students for suicide, which is actually much more common on campus than homicide. In fact, the JED Foundation has developed an excellent handbook,

Balancing Safety and Support on Campus: A Guide for Campus Teams, which can be downloaded free from their website, www.jedfoundation.org. This outlines how to form effective teams, how to create a "culture of caring" on campus, and how to address common obstacles. For a more in-depth discussion of behavioral intervention teams, see chapter 17.

In an increasingly digital age, new technologies and social media may create new ways to identify and approach at-risk students. One study used an interactive web-based questionnaire, which automatically triaged respondents into one of three risk categories, from high to low, and notified a screening counselor.[16] The counselor then posted an assessment for the student, inviting higher-risk students in for a face-to-face evaluation. Of the 572 students who fell into the high-risk category, 91% viewed the counselor's personalized assessment, 34% engaged in online dialogues with the counselor, 20% came for an in-person evaluation, and 15% entered treatment. Some students in this study clearly expressed their desire for treatment and extreme reluctance initially to come in person; some found the online communication a helpful first step. Although psychiatrists might be reluctant to engage in anonymous online dialogue with at-risk students for fear that identifying students but then being essentially unable to protect them puts both patient and doctor at risk, we might need to re-evaluate our practices through the lens of what is most likely to help the most students.

Student Emotional Well-Being

Looking toward the Future

Upon learning where I work, a first-year medical student recently told me, with some surprise, that at her Ivy League undergraduate school, one in five students supposedly used counseling services. She evidently considered this remarkably high. I asked whether it would it surprise her to learn that the majority of students had used the health center. Of course not, she said. I pointed out that just as "physical" health problems exist on a continuum, from the common cold to isolated injuries, such as a broken bone, to heart disease to cancer, so mental health difficulties encompass everything from adjusting to a new school in a new country to the grief of a broken heart to schizophrenia. She admitted that she, as both a student and a future health care provider, is still unintentionally stigmatizing mental health, and that the dichotomy between mind and body persists. But she rapidly recognized the issue and noted that her medical school does focus more on student well-being, including emotional well-being, and that she intends to learn to do that too.

Although the growth in numbers of students seeking mental health services during college and grad school may alarm university administrators from a resource management perspective, it presents wonderful opportunities. Emerging adults bring to college many of the problems they've grown up with—the lingering effects of domestic violence, combat, or other traumatic experiences;

the drinking habits or inattention to health that they've seen modeled at home or among their peers; and the tendencies to put extreme pressure on themselves in some areas while neglecting self-care or relationships. They bring their genetic vulnerabilities and complicated family dynamics. But they also bring great resilience and an eagerness to learn, and even the most depressed and seemingly hopeless among them step onto campus with some degree of hope that they are entering a new and better phase of life. They are at a crossroad. Their time on campus is a perfect window of opportunity to intervene and potentially change the course of their lives.

Clearly, the most effective interventions for this population are slightly different in some cases, and quite different in others, from ones we might employ with other populations and from those most psychiatrists learn during psychiatric residency. The most effective clinicians understand the emerging adult developmental framework, are familiar with generational trends, and strive to continually update their understanding of the multiple identities and diversity of backgrounds that students bring to school. Psychiatrists have much to offer emerging adult students, but not if we're narrowly focused on psychopharmacology or can't engage in sensitive, empathic, collaborative treatment planning. The most meaningful work will incorporate psychotherapeutic principles and techniques, many of which can be fit into either a brief framework or one of intermittent treatment.

The isolation faced by psychiatrists who worked with students as recently as 20 years ago is diminishing. Although many university counseling centers are still psychiatrically understaffed, there are trends toward growth. Some universities are starting new comprehensive counseling centers with plans to include psychiatric staffing. Others, such as Ohio State University, are offering psychiatric fellowship training in college mental health. The American Psychiatric Association recently re-established a College Mental Health Caucus. The University of Michigan hosts an annual "Depression on College Campuses" conference. And the National Network of Depression Centers formed a College Mental Health Task Force that is working toward facilitating research in this population as well as attempting to identify best practices.

New digital forums allow unprecedented communication among college psychiatrists, and we are raising questions, sharing best practices, and encouraging collaborations that will all improve the quality of the care we provide. Colleges are systematizing their referral networks, creating relationships with psychiatrists and other therapists in the communities around them who have experience and expertise treating emerging adults. Because of the range of issues students bring to us, best care will always involve an interdisciplinary approach, where psychiatrists, psychologists, social workers, and nurse practitioners collaborate and support one another, both on campus and off.

Healthcare is undergoing tremendous change, and mental health care in particular has become fragmented and often difficult to access across the United States. This can be particularly true for students who need mental health services. Attending productively to the mental health needs of this growing subset of tomorrow's adults will define not only their ability to flourish and succeed, but also to some extent the progress of our collective community. If we provide a range of services, including individual, group, and community programs, we will be in step with the goals of health care reform to focus on both prevention and optimizing outcomes. We need to empower students to recognize the range of problems they may encounter during their years in higher education, and then we need to do more research to improve our evidence base for what best works in this population.

Once we've done that, we will be on the path toward not just healthier universities, but also healthier future communities.

Notes

CHAPTER 1: Crisis on the College Campus?

1. Lewin, Tamar. (2011, Jan. 26). "Record Levels of Stress Found in College Freshmen." *New York Times.*

2. Higher Education Research Institute, "Incoming College Students Rate Emotional Health at Record Low, Annual Survey Finds," www.heri.ucla.edu/pr-display.php?prQry=55, accessed June 16, 2011.

3. Gallagher, Robert. National Survey of Counseling Center Directors, 2010. International Association of Counseling Services.

4. Sulzberger, A., & Gabriel, T. (2011, Jan. 13). "College's Policy on Troubled Students Raises Questions." *New York Times.*

5. Ibid.

6. Barr, V., et al. The Association for University and College Counseling Center Directors Annual Survey 2011.

7. Kay, Jerald, & Schwartz, Victor. (2010). *Mental health care in the college community.* West Sussex, UK: John Wiley & Sons.

8. Blanco, Carlos, et al. (2008). "Mental Health of College Students and Their Non-College-Attending Peers." *Archives of General Psychiatry, 65* (12): 1429–37.

9. National College Health Assessment, 2008.

10. American College Health Association—National College Health Assessment. (2008, March/April). "Spring 2007 Reference Group Data Report" (abridged). *Journal of American College Health, 56* (5): 469–79.

11. Gallagher, 2010.

12. Pleskac, T. J., et al. (2011). "A Detection Model of College Withdrawal." *Organizational Behavior and Human Decision Processes.* doi:10.1016/j.obhdp.2010.12.001.

CHAPTER 2: The Changing Face of the American University Student

1. National Center for Education Statistics. "Fast Facts: Enrollment." http://nces.ed.gov/fastfacts/display.asp?id=98, accessed June 27, 2011.

2. Ibid.

3. National Center for Education Statistics. "Post-Secondary Expectations of 12th Graders 2006." http://nces.ed.gov/programs/coe/indicator_ect.asp, accessed May 9, 2012.

4. Eisenberg, D., et al. (2007). "Prevalence and Correlates of Depression, Anxiety and Suicidality among University Students." *American Journal of Orthopsychiatry, 77* (4): 534–42.

5. NASPA. (2008). Profile of Today's College Student. Survey. www.naspa.org/divctr/research/profile/survey.cfm.

6. Young, Amanda. (2011, Winter). "Gay Students: The Latest Outreach Target at Many Colleges." *Journal of College Admission*, 38–39.

7. Kearney, Lisa, Draper, Matthew, & Baron, Augustine. (2005). "Counseling Utilization by Ethnic Minority College Students." *Cultural Diversity and Ethnic Minority Psychology*, 11 (3): 272–85.

8. Mitchell, Sharon, Greenwood, Andrea, & Guglielmi, Maggie. (2007). "Utilization of Counseling Services: Comparing International and U.S. College Students." *Journal of College Counseling*, 10, 117–29.

9. Tochkov, K., Levine, L., & Sanaka, A. (2010). "Variation in the Prediction of Cross-Cultural Adjustment by Asian-Indian Students in the United States." *College Student Journal, 44* (3): 677–89.

10. Fischer, Karin. (2011, April 3). "Commerce Dept. Takes Greater Role in Promoting U.S. Higher Education Overseas." *Chronicle of Higher Education.*

11. "International-Student Recruitment Debate: 6 Views on Agents." (2011, June 16). Commentary in *Chronicle of Higher Education.*

12. Aslanian, C., & Giles, N. G. (2009, Aug. 12). "Hindsight, Insight, Foresight: Understanding Adult Learning Trends to Predict Future Opportunities." www.education dynamics.com/Market-Research/White-Papers.aspx.

13. Hadley, W. M. (2011). "College Students with Disabilities: A Student Development Perspective." *New Directions for Higher Education, 77–81.*

14. "VA Web Site Helps College Counselors Aid Veterans." (2009, June 8). *Mental Health Weekly Digest, 162.*

CHAPTER 3: Generational Issues on Campus

1. Howe, Neil, & Strauss, William. (2003). *Millennials go to college.* Washington, D.C.: American Association of Collegiate Registrars.

2. Twenge, Jean, & Campbell, Stacy. (2008). "Generational Differences in Psychological Traits and Their Impact on the Workplace." *Journal of Managerial Psychology, 23* (8): 862–77.

3. Howe & Strauss, 2003.

4. Pryor, J. H., DeAngelo, L., Palucki Blake, L., Hurtado, S., & Tran, S. (2011). *The American freshman: National norms fall 2011.* Los Angeles: Higher Education Research Institute, UCLA.

5. Ibid.

6. Twenge & Campbell, 2008.

7. Hoover, Eric. (2009, Oct. 11). "The Millennial Muddle: How Stereotyping Students Became a Thriving Industry, and a Bundle of Contradictions." *Chronicle of Higher Education.*

8. Bonner, F. A., Lewis, C. W., Bowman-Perrott, L., & Hill-Jackson, V. (2009). "Definition, Identification, Identity and Culture: A Unique Alchemy Impacting the Success of Gifted African American Millennial Males in School." *Journal for the Education of the Gifted 33* (2): 176–202.

9. Twenge & Campbell, 2008. Trzesniewski, K. H., Donnellan, M. B., & Robins,

R. W. (2008). "Do Today's Young People Really Think They Are So Extraordinary? An Examination of Secular Changes in Narcissism and Self-Enhancement." *Psychological Science, 19* (2): 181–8.

10. Zill, Nicholas, & Robinson, John P. (1995, April). "The Generation X Difference." *American Demographics, 17* (4): 24–33.

11. Borges, N. J., Manuel, R. S., Elam, C. L., & Jones, B. J. (2006, June). "Comparing Millennial and Generation X Medical Students at One Medical School." *Academic Medicine, 81* (6): 571–76.

12. Zill & Robinson, 1995.

13. Datatel 2006 College Parent Survey summary, *LifeCourse Associates*, https://store.lifecourse.com/products/2/Millennials+Go+To+College.html?ref=alt.

14. Twenge & Campbell, 2008.

15. Wesner, Marilyn S., & Miller, Tammy. (2008, Fall). "Boomers and Millennials Have Much in Common." *Organization Development Journal, 26* (3): 89.

16. Twenge & Campbell, 2008.

17. Howe, Neil, & Strauss, William. (2007, Nov.). "Helicopter Parents in the Workplace." *New Paradigm Learning Corporation.*

18. Arnett, Jeffrey. (2000, May). "Emerging Adulthood: A Theory of Development from the Late Teens to the Twenties." *American Psychologist, 55* (5): 469–80.

19. Ibid.

20. Luna, B. (2009). "The Maturation of Cognitive Control and the Adolescent Brain." In F. Aboitiz & D. Cosmelli (Eds.), *Attention to goal-directed behavior* (pp. 249–74). Berlin: Springer-Verlag.

21. Bennett, C. M., & Baird, A. A. (2006). "Anatomical Changes in the Emerging Adult Brain: A Voxel-Based Morphometry Study." *Human Brain Mapping, 27,* 766–77.

22. Arnett, Jeffrey J., & Tanner, Jennifer L. (2009). "The Emergence of 'Emerging Adulthood.'" In A. Furlong (Ed.), *Handbook of youth and young adulthood* (pp. 39–45). London and New York: Routledge, 2009.

23. Ibid.

CHAPTER 4: The Psychiatrist's Role in College Mental Health

1. Barreira, P., & Snider, M. (2010). "History of College Counseling and Mental Health Services and Role of the Community Mental Health Model." In J. Kay & V. Schwartz (Eds.), *Mental health care in the college community* (pp. 21–31). Oxford: Wiley & Sons.

2. Eisenberg, D., & Chung, H. (2012). "Adequacy of Depression Treatment among College Students in the United States." *General Hospital Psychiatry, 34* (3): 213–20.

3. Ibid.

CHAPTER 5: Sleep Problems on Campus

1. American College Health Association. (2009). *American College Health Association–National College Health Assessment II: Reference group executive summary spring 2009.* Linthicum, MD: American College Health Association.

2. Brown, F. C., Buboltz, W. C., & Soper, B. (2002, Spring). "Relationship of Sleep

Hygiene Awareness, Sleep Hygiene Practices, and Sleep Quality in University Students." *Behavioral Medicine, 28,* 33–38.

3. Reissig, C. J., Strain, E. C., & Griffiths, R. R. (2009, Jan. 1). "Caffeinated Energy Drinks—A Growing Problem." *Drug and Alcohol Dependence, 99* (1–3): 1–10.

4. O'Brien, M. C., McCoy, T. P., Rhodes, S. D., Wagoner, A., & Wolfson, M. (2008, May). "Caffeinated Cocktails: Energy Drink Consumption, High-Risk Drinking, and Alcohol-Related Consequences among College Students." *Academic Emergency Medicine, 15* (5): 453–60.

5. Wilson, S. J., Nutt, D. J., Alford, C., Argyropoulos, S. V., Baldwin, D. S., Bateson, A. N., Britton, T. C., Crowe, C., Dijk, D.-J., Espie, C. A., Gringras, P., Hajak, G., Idzikowski, C., Krystal, A. D., Nash, J. R., Selsick, H., Sharpley, A. L., & Wade, A. G. (2010, Sept.). "British Association for Psychopharmacology consensus statement on evidence-based treatment of insomnia, parasomnias and circadian rhythm disorders." *Journal of Psychopharmacology Online First,* http://jop.sagepub.com/content/early/2010/08/31/0269881110379307.

6. Carney, C. E., Edinger, J. D., Meyer, B., Lindman, L., & Istre, T. (2006). "Daily Activities and Sleep Quality in College Students." *Chronobiology International, 23* (3): 623–37; and Brown et al., 2002.

7. Carney et al., 2006.

8. Wilson et al., 2010.

9. Carney, C. E., & Waters, W. F. (2006). "Effects of a Structured Problem-Solving Procedure on Pre-Sleep Cognitive Arousal in College Students with Insomnia." *Behavioral Sleep Medicine, 4* (1): 13–28.

10. Ong, J. C., Shapiro, S. L., & Manber, R. (2008). "Combining Mindfulness Meditation with Cognitive-Behavior Therapy for Insomnia: A Treatment-Development Study." *Behavior Therapy, 39,* 171–82.

11. Rogers, H., & Maytan, M. (2012). *Mindfulness for the next generation.* New York: Oxford University Press, p. 51.

12. Wilson et al., 2010.

13. Brown, F., Soper B., & Buboltz Jr., W. (2001, Sept.). "Prevalence of Delayed Sleep Phase Syndrome in University Students." *College Student Journal* [serial online], *35* (3): 472. Available from Academic Search Premier, Ipswich, MA.

14. Brown, F. C., Buboltz, W. C., & Soper, B. (2006). "Development and Evaluation of the Sleep Treatment and Education Program for Students (STEPS)." *Journal of American College Health, 54* (4): 231–37.

15. Lack, L. C., & Wright, H. R. (2007). "Treating Chronobiological Components of Chronic Insomnia." *Sleep Medicine, 8,* 637–44.

CHAPTER 6: Alcohol on Campus

1. Hingson, R. W., Heeren, T., & Winter, M. R. (2006, Sept.). "Age of Alcohol-Dependence Onset: Associations with Severity of Dependence and Seeking Treatment." *Pediatrics, 118* (3): e755–e763.

2. Wechsler, H., & Nelson, T. F. (2008, July). "What We Have Learned From the Harvard School of Public Health College Alcohol Study: Focusing Attention on Col-

lege Student Alcohol Consumption and the Environmental Conditions That Promote It." *Journal of Studies on Alcohol and Drugs, 69* (4): 481–90.

3. Hingson, R. W., Zha, W., & Weitzman, E. R. (2009). "Magnitude of and Trends in Alcohol-Related Mortality and Morbidity among U.S. College Students Ages 18–24, 1998–2005." *Journal of Studies on Alcohol and Drugs,* Supplement 16, 12–20.

4. Ibid.

5. O'Malley, P. M., & Johnson, L. D. (2002). "Epidemiology of Alcohol and Other Drug Use among American College Students." *Journal of Studies on Alcohol and Drugs,* Supplement 14, 23–39.

6. National Institute on Alcohol and Alcohol Abuse. (2002, Oct.). *Alcohol Alert, 58.* http://pubs.niaaa.nih.gov/publications/aa58.htm.

7. O'Malley & Johnson, 2002.

8. NIAAA, 2002.

9. Slutske, W. S. (2005). "Alcohol Use Disorders among US College Students and Their Non–College-Attending Peers." *Archives of General Psychiatry, 62,* 321–27.

10. Wechsler & Nelson, 2008.

11. Hoeppner, B. B., Paskausky, A. L., Jackson, K. M., & Barnett, N. P. (2013). "Sex Differences in College Student Adherence to NIAAA Drinking Guidelines." *Alcoholism: Clinical and Experimental Research.* doi:10.1111/acer.12159.

12. Paschall, M. J., Antin, T., Ringwalt, C. L., & Saltz, R. F. (2011). "Effects of AlcoholEdu for College on Alcohol-Related Problems among Freshmen: A Randomized Multicampus Trial." *Journal of Studies on Alcohol and Drugs, 7,* 642–50.

13. NREPP. "Brief Alcohol Screening and Interventions for College Students (BASICS)." http://nrepp.samhsa.gov/ViewIntervention.aspx?id=124, accessed Sept. 12, 2011.

14. Perkins, H. W. (2002). "Social Norms and the Prevention of Alcohol Misuse in Collegiate Contexts." *Journal of Studies on Alcohol and Drugs,* Supplement 14, 164–72.

15. Carey, K. B., Scott-Sheldon, L. A., Carey, M. P., & DeMartini, K. S. (2007, Nov.). "Individual-Level Interventions to Reduce College Student Drinking: A Meta-analytic Review." *Addictive Behaviors, 32* (11): 2469–94.

16. Brady, K. T., & Verduin, M. L. (2005). "Pharmacotherapy of Comorbid Mood, Anxiety, and Substance Use Disorders." *Substance Use & Misuse, 40,* 2021–41.

17. Dundon, W. D., & Pettinatti, H. M. (2011, June). "Comorbid Depression and Alcohol Dependence: New Approaches to Dual Therapy Challenges and Progress." *Psychiatric Times, 28* (6): 49.

18. Lamps, C. A., Sood, A. B., & Sood, R. (2008). "Youth with Substance Abuse and Comorbid Mental Health Disorders." *Current Psychiatry Reports, 10,* 265–71; and Dundon & Pettinatti, 2011.

19. Ostacher, M. J. (2007). "Comorbid Alcohol and Substance Abuse Dependence in Depression: Impact on the Outcome of Antidepressant Treatment." *Psychiatric Clinics of North America, 30* (1): 69–76.

20. Bukstein, O. G., Clark, D. B., & Cornelius, J. R. (2006, Oct. 1). "Treating Adolescents with Major Depression and an Alcohol Use Disorder." *Psychiatric Times, 23* (11): 32.

21. Dundon & Pettinatti, 2011.

22. Frye, M. A., & Salloum, I. M. (2006). "Bipolar Disorder and Comorbid Alcoholism: Prevalence Rate and Treatment Considerations." *Bipolar Disorders, 8,* 677–85. doi:10.1111/j.1399-5618.2006.00370.

23. "Survey: Students Don't Associate Untreated Bipolar Disorder with Risks." (2003, Nov. 10). *Mental Health Weekly Digest.* Retrieved from HighBeam Research, www.highbeam.com/doc/1G1-109912353.html.

24. Frye & Salloum, 2006.

CHAPTER 7: Non-alcohol Substance Abuse on Campus

1. Buckner, J. D., Ecker, A. H., & Cohen, A. S. (2010). "Mental Health Problems and Interest in Marijuana Treatment among Marijuana-Using College Students." *Addictive Behaviors, 35,* 826–33.

2. Meier, M. H., Caspi, A., & Ambler, A., et al. (2012). "Persistent Cannabis Users Show Neuropsychological Decline from Childhood to Midlife." *Proceedings of the National Academy of Sciences,* early edition, 1–8.

3. Carpenter, K. M., McDowell, D., Brooks, D. J., Cheng, W. Y., & Levin, F. R. (2009). "A Preliminary Trial: Double-Blind Comparison of Nefazodone, Bupropion-SR and Placebo in the Treatment of Cannabis Dependence." *American Journal on Addictions, 18,* 53–64. Trezza, V., Cuomo, V., & Vanderschuren, L. J. "Cannabis and the Developing Brain: Insights from Behavior." (2008). *European Journal of Pharmacology, 585* (2–3): 441–52.

4. Milin, R., Manion, I., Dare, G., & Walker, S. (2008). "Prospective Assessment of Cannabis Withdrawal in Adolescents with Cannabis Dependence: A Pilot Study." *Journal of the American Academy of Child Adolescent Psychiatry, 42* (2): 174–79.

5. Carpenter et al., 2009.

6. Milin et al., 2008.

7. Lundqvist, T. (2005). "Cognitive Consequences of Cannabis Use: Comparison with Abuse of Stimulants and Heroin with Regard to Attention, Memory and Executive Functions." *Pharmacology, Biochemistry and Behavior, 81* (2): 319–30.

8. Pierre, J. M. (2011). "Cannabis, Synthetic Cannabinoids, and Psychosis Risk: What the Evidence Says." *Current Psychiatry, 10* (9): 49–58.

9. Buckner et al., 2010.

10. Pierre, 2011.

11. Ibid.

12. Rostain, A. L. (2006). "Addressing the Misuse and Abuse of Stimulant Medications on College Campuses." *Current Psychiatry Reports, 8,* 335–336.

13. Volkow, N. D. (2006). "Stimulant Medications: How to Minimize Their Reinforcing Effects." *American Journal of Psychiatry, 163,* 3.

14. Greely, H. (2008). Towards Responsible Use Of Cognitive-Enhancing Drugs by the Healthy. *Nature, 456* (7223): 702–5.

15. Rosenfield, D., Hebert, P. C., & Stanbrook, M. B. (2011). "Time to Address Stimulant Abuse on Our Campuses." *CMAJ, 183* (12): 1345.

16. Rostain, 2006.

17. Johnston, L. D., O'Malley, P. M., Bachman, J. G., & Schulenberg, J. E. (2011). *Monitoring the future national survey results on drug use, 1975–2010: Volume II, College*

students and adults ages 19–50. Ann Arbor: Institute for Social Research, University of Michigan.

18. DeMaria, P. A., Sterling, R. C., Risler, R., & Frank, J. (2010). "Using Buprenorphine to Treat Opiod-Dependent University Students." *Journal of Addiction Medicine, 4,* 236–42.

19. Johnston et al., 2011.

20. Ibid.

21. Arria, Amelia M., et al. (2006). "Evidence for Significant Polydrug Use among Ecstasy-Using College Students." *Journal of American College Health, 55* (2): 99–104.

22. Ahern, N. R., & Greenberg, C. S. (2011). Psychoactive Herb Use and Youth: A Closer Look at Salvia Divinorum. *Journal of Psychosocial Nursing & Mental Health Services, 49* (8): 16–19. doi:10.3928/02793695-20110705-05.

23. Ross, E. A., Watson, M., & Goldberger, B. (2011). "'Bath Salts' Intoxication." *New England Journal of Medicine, 365* (10): 967–68.

CHAPTER 8: Loneliness and Relationships on Campus

1. Dellinger-Ness, L. A., & Handler, L. (2007, Fall). "Self-Injury, Gender, and Loneliness among College Students." *Journal of College Counseling, 10* (2): 142.

2. Wei, M., Russell, D. W., & Zakalik, R. A. (2005). "Adult Attachment, Social Self-Efficacy, Self-Disclosure, Loneliness, and Subsequent Depression for Freshman College Students: A Longitudinal Study." *Journal of Counseling Psychology, 52* (4): 602–614.

3. Ibid.

4. Owen, J. J., et al. (2010). "'Hooking Up' among College Students: Demographic and Psychosocial Correlates." *Archives of Sexual Behavior, 39,* 653–63.

5. Ibid.

6. Bradshaw, C., Kahn, A. S., & Saville, B. K. (2010). "To Hook Up or Date: Which Gender Benefits?" *Sex Roles, 62,* 661–69.

7. Owen et al., 2010.

8. Bradshaw et al., 2010.

9. Owen, J., Fincham, F. D., & Moore, J. (2011). "Short-Term Prospective Study of Hooking Up among College Students." *Archives of Sexual Behavior, 40,* 331–41.

10. Asher, S. R., & Weeks, M. S. (2012). *Social relationships, academic engagement, and well-being in college: Executive summary of findings from the Duke Social Relationships Project.* http://sites.duke.edu/dsrp.

11. Bogle, K. A. (2008). *Hooking up: Sex, dating and relationships on campus.* New York: New York University Press.

12. Asher & Weeks, 2012.

13. "New mtvU—Associated Press Study Examines College Students' Mental Health and Relationship with Technology." (2010, Oct. 18). *Mental Health Weekly Digest,* 141.

14. Moreno, M. A., et al. (2011). "Feeling Bad on Facebook: Depression Disclosures by College Students on a Social Networking Site." *Depression and Anxiety, 28,* 447–55.

15. Kuss, D. J., & Griffiths, M. D. (2011). "Online Social Networking and Addiction— A Review of the Psychological Literature." *International Journal of Environmental Research and Public Health, 8,* 3528–52.

16. Heisel, M., Flett, G., & Hewitt. P. (2003). "Social Hopelessness and College Student Suicide." *Archives of Suicide Research, 7,* 221–35.

17. Ibid.

18. Furr, S. R., et al. (2001). "Suicide and Depression among College Students: A Decade Later." *Professional Psychology: Research and Practice, 32* (1): 97–100.

19. Asher & Weeks, 2012.

CHAPTER 9: Perfectionism

1. Burns, D. D. (1980). "The Perfectionist's Script for Self-Defeat." *Psychology Today,* 34–51.

2. Kutlesa, N., & Arthur, N. (2008). "Overcoming Negative Aspects of Perfectionism through Group Treatment." *Journal of Rational-Emotive & Cognitive-Behavior Therapy, 26,* 134–54.

3. Klibert, J., Langhinrichsen-Rohling, J., & Saito, M. (2005). "Adaptive and Maladaptive Aspects of Self-Oriented versus Socially Prescribed Perfectionism." *Journal College Student Development, 46* (2): 141–56.

4. O'Connor, R. C. (2007). "The Relations between Perfectionism and Suicidality: A Systematic Review." *Suicide & Life-Threatening Behavior, 37* (6): 698–714.

5. Bieling, P. J., Israeli, A. L., & Anthony, M. M. (2004). "Is Perfectionism Good, Bad, or Both? Examining Models of the Perfectionism Construct." *Personality and Individual Differences, 36* (6): 1373–85.

6. Rice, K. G., et al. (2012). "Self-Critical Perfectionism, Acculturative Stress and Depression among International Students." *Counseling Psychologist, 40* (4): 575–600.

7. Ibid.

8. Sherry, S. N., et al. (2004). "Self-Oriented and Socially Prescribed Perfectionism in the Eating Disorder Inventory Perfectionism Subscale." *International Journal of Eating Disorders, 35,* 69–79.

9. Klibert et al., 2005.

10. Ibid.

11. Kutlesa & Arthur, 2008.

CHAPTER 10: Clash of Cultures: International Students

1. Mori, S. (2000, Spring). "Addressing the Mental Health Concerns of International Students." *Journal of Counseling and Development, 78* (2): 137.

2. Nilsson, J. E., Berkel, L. A., Flores, L. Y., & Lucas, M. S. (2004). "Utilization Rate and Presenting Concerns of International Students at a University Counseling Center: Implications for Outreach Programming." *Journal of College Student Psychotherapy,* 19 (2): 49–59. Yakushko, O., Davidson, M., & Sanford-Martens, T. (2008). "Seeking Help in a Foreign Land: International Students' Use Patterns for a U.S. University Counseling Center." *Journal of College Counseling, 11,* 6–18.

3. Mitchell, S. L., Greenwood, A. K., & Guglielmi, M. C. (2007). "Utilization of Counseling Services: Comparing International and U.S. College Students." *Journal of College Counseling, 10,* 117–29.

4. Yakushko et al., 2008.

5. Levine, Lisa, Sanaka, Amritha, & Tochkov, Karin. (2010). "Variation in the Prediction of Cross-Cultural Adjustment by Asian-Indian Students in the United States." *College Student Journal, 44* (3): 677.

6. Dipeolu, A., Kang, J., & Cooper, C. (2007). "Support Group for International Students: A Counseling Center's Experience." *Journal of College Student Psychotherapy, 22* (1): 63.

7. Ibid.

8. Yoo, S. K., & Skovholt, T. M. (2001). "Cross-Cultural Examination of Depression Expression and Help-Seeking Behavior: A Comparative Study of American and Korean College Students." *Journal of College Counseling, 4,* 10–19.

9. Essandoh, Pius. (1995). "Counseling Issues with African College Students in U.S. Colleges and Universities." *Counseling Psychologist, 23,* 348.

CHAPTER 11: Clash of Cultures: LGBT Students

1. Rankin, S. R. (2003). *Campus climate for gay, lesbian, bisexual, and transgender people: A national perspective.* New York, NY: The National Gay and Lesbian Task Force Policy Institute.

2. Schmidt, C. K., et al. (2011). "Perceived Discrimination and Social Support: The Influences on Career Development and College Adjustment of LGBT College Students." *Journal of Career Development, 38* (4): 293–309.

3. Grossman, A. H., & D'Augell, A. R. (2007). "Transgender Youth and Life-Threatening Behaviors." *Suicide and Life-Threatening Behavior, 37* (5): 527–37.

4. Sanlo, R. (2004–2005). "Lesbian, Gay and Bisexual College Students: Risk, Resiliency and Retention." *Journal of College Student Retention, 6* (1): 97–110.

5. Cohen, K. M. (2006). "Sexual Concerns." In P. A. Grayson & P. W. Meilman (Eds.), *College mental health practice* (pp. 228–36). New York: Routledge.

6. Else-Quest, N. (2008). "Gender and Sexual Orientation." In S. F. Davis & W. Buskist (Eds.), *21st century psychology: A reference handbook* (pp. II-460–II-470). Thousand Oaks, CA: Sage.

7. Spitzer, R. L. (2012). "Spitzer Reassesses His 2003 Study of Reparative Therapy of Homosexuality." *Archives of Sexual Behavior, 41, 757.*

8. "Lambda Legal Applauds Law Banning 'Reparative Therapy' for California Minors." (2012, Aug. 29). *Targeted News Service.*

9. Bartoli, E., & Gillam, A. (2008). "Continuing to Depolarize the Debate on Sexual Orientation and Religion: Identity and the Therapeutic Process." *Professional Psychology: Research and Practice, 39* (2): 202–9.

10. Rankin, 2003.

11. WPATH De-Psychopatholisation Statement, released May 26, 2010. www.wpath .org.

12. Effrig, J. C., Bieschke, K. J., & Locke, B. D. (2011). "Victimization and Psychological Distress in Transgender College Students." *Journal of College Counseling, 14,* 143–57.

13. Institute of Medicine. (2011). *The health of lesbian, gay, bisexual, and transgender people: Building a foundation for better understanding.* Washington, D.C.: National Academies Press.

14. *Gay and Lesbian Alliance Against Defamation (GLAAD) media guide 2010.*

15. UC Berkeley Gender Equity Resource Center, http://geneq.berkeley.edu/lgbt _resources_definiton_of_terms, accessed Sept. 14, 2012.

16. Effrig et al., 2011.

17. Grossman & D'Augell, 2007.

18. Effrig et al., 2011.

19. McKinney, J. S. (2005). "On the Margins: A Study of the Experiences of Transgender College Students," *Journal of Gay & Lesbian Issues in Education, 3* (1): 63–75.

20. World Professional Association for Transgender Health. (2011). "Standards of Care for the Health of Transsexual, Transgender, and Gender Nonconforming People." Version 7. *International Journal of Transgenderism, 13,* 165–232.

CHAPTER 12: Disordered Eating

1. Krahn, D. D., Kurth, C. L., Gomberg, E., & Drewnowski, A. (2005). "Pathological Dieting and Alcohol Use in College Women—A Continuum of Behaviors." *Eating Behaviors, 6,* 43–52.

2. American Psychiatric Association. (2000). *Diagnostic and statistical manual of mental disorders,* 4th ed., text revision. Washington, D.C.: American Psychiatric Association.

3. Yeh, H.-W., Tzeng, N.-S., Chu, H., Chou, Y., Lu, R., O'Brien, A. P., Chang, Y., Hsieh, C., & Chou, K. (2009). "The Risk of Eating Disorders among Female Undergraduates in Taiwan." *Archives of Psychiatric Nursing, 23* (6): 430–40.

4. Beekley, M. D., Byrne, R., Yavorek, T., Kidd, K., Wolff, J., & Johnson, M. (2009). "Incidence, Prevalence, and Risk of Eating Disorder Behaviors in Military Academy Cadets." *Military Medicine, 174* (6): 637–41.

5. Feldman, M. B., & Meyer, I. H. (2010). "Comorbidity and Age of Onset of Eating Disorders in Gay Men, Lesbians, and Bisexuals." *Psychiatry Research, 180* (2): 126–31.

6. Eisenberg, D., Nicklett, E. J., Roeder, K., & Kirz, N. E. (2011). "Eating Disorder Symptoms among College Students: Prevalence, Persistence, Correlates, and Treatment-Seeking." *Journal of American College Health, 59* (8): 700–7.

7. Ibid.

8. Berg, K. C., Frazier, P., & Sherr, L. (2009). "Changes in Eating Disorder Attitudes and Behavior in College Women: Prevalence and Predictors." *Eating Behaviors, 10,* 137–42.

9. Krahn et al., 2005.

10. Treasure, J., Claudino, A. M., & Zucker, N. (2010). "Eating Disorders." *Lancet, 375,* 583–93.

11. Krahn et al., 2005.

12. Kelly-Weeder, S., & Edwards, E. (2011). "Co-occurring Binge Eating and Binge Drinking in College Women." *Journal for Nurse Practitioners, 7* (3): 207–13.

13. Whitlock, J., Eckenrode, J., & Silverman, D. (2006). "Self-Injurious Behaviors in a College Population." *Pediatrics, 117,* 1939.

14. Wilcox, H. C., Arria. A. M., & Caldeira, K. M., et al. (2012). "Longitudinal Predictors of Past-Year Non-suicidal Self-Injury and Motives among College Students." *Psychological Medicine, 42* (4): 717–26.

15. APA. *DSM-5 Development*. www.dsm5.org, accessed June 23, 2012.

16. Ferriter, C., & Ray, L. A. (2011). "Binge Eating and Binge Drinking: An Integrative Review." *Eating Behaviors, 12*, 99–107.

17. Yager, J., Kurtzman, F., Landsverk, J., & Wiesmeier, E. (1988). "Behaviors and Attitudes Related to Eating Disorders in Homosexual Male College Students." *American Journal of Psychiatry, 145*, 495–97. Carper, T. L., Negy, C., & Tantleff-Dunn, S. (2010). "Relations among Media Influence, Body Image, Eating Concerns, and Sexual Orientation in Men: A Preliminary Investigation." *Body Image, 7* (4): 301–9.

18. Carper et al., 2010.

19. Alpert, E. (2013, June 13). "Eating Disorders Plague Teenage Boys, Too." *Los Angeles Times*.

20. Feldman & Meyer, 2010.

21. Franko, D. L., Becker, A. E., Thomas, J. J., & Herzog, D. B. (2007). "Cross-Ethnic Differences in Eating Disorder Symptoms and Related Distress." *International Journal of Eating Disorders, 40*, 156–64.

22. Berg et al., 2009.

23. Spillane, N. S., Boerner, L. M., Anderson, K. G., & Smith, G. T. (2004). "Comparability of the Eating Disorder Inventory-2 Between Women and Men." *Assessment, 11* (1): 85–93.

24. Treasure, J., Whitaker, W., Whitney, J., & Schmidt, U. (2005). "Working with Families of Adults with Anorexia Nervosa." *Journal of Family Therapy, 27* (2): 158–70.

25. Treasure, Claudino et al., 2010.

26. Ibid. American Psychiatric Association. (2006). *Practice guideline for the treatment of patients with eating disorders*, 3rd ed. Arlington, VA: APA.

27. APA, *Practice Guideline*, 2006.

CHAPTER 13: Difficulty Concentrating

1. Rabiner, D. L., Anastopoulos, A. D., Costello, E. J., Hoyle, R. H., McCabe, S. E., & Swartzwelder, H. S. (2009). "Motives and Perceived Consequences of Nonmedical ADHD Medication Use by College Students: Are Students Treating Themselves for Attention Problems?" *Journal of Attention Disorders, 13*, 259–70. Greeley, H., et al. (2008). "Towards Responsible Use of Cognitive-Enhancing Drugs by the Healthy." *Nature, 456* (11): 702–5.

2. Rabiner et al., 2009.

3. Wolf, L. E., Simkowitz, P., & Carlson, H. (2009). "College Students with Attention-Deficit/Hyperactivity Disorder." *Current Psychiatry Reports, 11*, 415–21.

4. Rabiner et al., 2009.

5. DuPaul, G. J., Weyandt, L. L, O'Dell, S. M., & Varejao, M. (2009). "College Students with ADHD: Current Status and Future Directions." *Journal of Attention Disorders, 13*, 234–50.

6. Glutting, J. J., Sheslow, D., & Adams, W. (2002). *CARE College ADHD response evaluation manual*. Wilmington, DE: Wide Range.

7. Nelson, J. M., & Gregg, N. (2012). "Depression and Anxiety among Transitioning Adolescents and College Students with ADHD, Dyslexia or Comorbid ADHD/

Dyslexia." *Journal of Attention Disorders, 16,* 244. Originally published online October 26, 2010. doi:10.1177/1087054710385783.

8. DuPaul et al., 2009.

9. Wolf et al., 2009.

10. Kessler, R. C., Adler, L., Ames, M., Demler, O., Faraone, S., Hiripi, E., Howess, M. J., Jin, R., Secnik, K., Spencer, T, Ustun, T. B., & Walters, E. (2005). "The World Health Organization Adult ADHD Self-Report Scale (ASRS): A Short Screening Scale for Use in the General Population." *Psychological Medicine, 35,* 245–56. doi:10.1017/S0033291704002892.

11. Garnier-Dykstra, L. M., Pinchevsky, G. M., Caldeira, K. M., Vincent, K. B., & Arria, A. M. (2010). "Self-Reported Adult Attention-Deficit/Hyperactivity Disorder Symptoms among College Students." *Journal of American College Health, 59* (2): 133–36.

12. Graham, N. A., DuPont, R. L., Gold, M. S., & Wilens, T. E. (2007). "Symptoms of ADHD or Marijuana Use? Dr. Wilens Replies." *American Journal of Psychiatry, 164* (6): 973–74. Wolf et al., 2009.

13. Pope, H. G., & Yurgelun-Todd, D. (1996). "The Residual Cognitive Effects of Heavy Marijuana Use in College Students." *Journal of the American Medical Association, 275,* 521–27.

14. Graham et al., 2007.

15. Rooney, M., et al. (2012). "Substance Use in College Students with ADHD." *Journal of Attention Disorders, 16,* 221. Originally published online Feb. 2, 2011. doi:10.1177/1087054710392536.

16. Wilens, T. E. (2006). Attention-Deficit Hyperactivity Disorder and Substance Use Disorders. *American Journal of Psychiatry, 163* (12): 2059–63. Pope & Yurgelun-Todd, 1996.

17. DuPaul et al., 2009.

18. Greeley et al., 2008.

19. Schwartz, A. (2013, Feb. 2). "Drowned in a Stream of Prescriptions." *New York Times.*

20. Becker-Mattes, A., Mattes, J. A., Abikoff, H., & Brandt, L. (1985). "State-Dependent Learning in Hyperactive Children Receiving Methylphenidate." *American Journal of Psychiatry, 142,* 455–59.

21. Sanday, L., Patti, C. L., Zanin, K. A., Tufik, S., & Frussa-Filho, R. (2012). "Amphetamine-Induced Memory Impairment in a Discriminative Avoidance Task Is State-Dependent in Mice." *International Journal of Neuropsychopharmacology,* available on CJO2012. doi:10.1017/S1461145712000296.

22. Wood, S. C., & Anagnostaras, S. G. (2009). "Memory and Psychostimulants: Modulation of Pavlovian Fear Conditioning by Amphetamine in C57BL/6 Mice." *Psychopharmacology, 202,* 197–206.

23. Wilens, 2006.

24. DuPaul, G. J., Weyandt, L. L., Rossi, J. S., Vilardo, B. A., O'Dell, S. M., Carson, K. M., Verdi, G., & Swentosky, A. (2012). "Double-Blind, Placebo-Controlled, Crossover Study of the Efficacy and Safety of Lisdexamfetamine Dimesylate in College Students with ADHD." *Journal of Attention Disorders, 16* (3): 202–20.

25. DuPaul et al., 2009.

CHAPTER 14: Anxiety

1. American College Health Association. (2011). *American College Health Association–National College Health Assessment Survey: Reference group executive summary, fall 2011.* Linthicum, MD: American College Health Association.

2. Benton, S. A., Robertson, J. M., Tseng, W. C., Newton, F. B., & Benton, S. L. (2003). "Changes in Counseling Center Client Problems across 13 Years." *Professional Psychology: Research and Practice, 34,* 66–72.

3. Cooper, Stewart E. (Ed.). (2005). "Evidence-Based Practice for Anxiety Disorders in College Mental Health." In *Evidence-based psychotherapy practice in college mental health* (pp. 33–48). Philadelphia, PA: Haworth Press. Anxiety and Depression Association of America, www.adaa.org.

4. Eisenberg, D., et al. (2007). "Prevalence and Correlates of Depression, Anxiety and Suicidality among University Students." *American Journal of Orthopsychiatry, 77* (4): 534–42.

5. Ruscio, A. M. (2002). "Delimiting the Boundaries of Generalized Anxiety Disorder: Differentiating High Worriers with and without GAD." *Journal of Anxiety Disorders, 16,* 377–400.

6. Raj, B. A., & Sheehan, D. V. (2001). "Social Anxiety Disorder." *Medical Clinics of North America, 85* (3): 711–33.

7. Stewart, D., & Mandrusiak, M. (2007). "Social Phobia in College Students: A Developmental Perspective." *Journal of College Student Psychotherapy, 22* (2): 49–65.

8. Hazlett-Stevens, H., Craske, M. G., Mayer, E. A., Chang, L., & Naliboff, B. D. (2003). "Prevalence of Irritable Bowel Syndrome among University Students: The Roles of Worry, Neuroticism, Anxiety Sensitivity and Visceral Anxiety." *Journal of Psychosomatic Research, 55,* 501–15.

9. Bostwick, W. B., Boyd, C. J., Hughes, T. L., & McCabe, S. E. (2010). "Dimensions of Sexual Orientation and the Prevalence of Mood and Anxiety Disorders in the United States." *American Journal of Public Health, 100* (3): 468–75.

10. National Institute for Mental Health. "Obsessive Compulsive Disorder among Adults." www.nimh.nih.gov/statistics/1OCD_ADULT.shtml, accessed July 9, 2012.

11. Cowley, Deborah. (2011, June 13). "Is OCD an Anxiety Disorder?" *Journal Watch Psychiatry.*

12. Sulkowski, M. L., Mariaskin, A., & Storch, E. A. (2011). "Obsessive-Compulsive Spectrum Disorder Symptoms in College Students." *Journal of American College Health, 59* (5): 342–48.

13. Tech, M. J., Lucas, J. A., & Nelson, P. (1989). "Nonclinical Panic in College Students: An Investigation of Prevalence and Symptomatology." *Journal of Abnormal Psychology, 98* (3): 300–306.

14. Frazer, P., Anders, S., Sulani, P., Tomich, P., Tennen, H., Park, C., & Tashiro, T. (2009). "Traumatic Events among Undergraduate Students: Prevalence and Associated Symptoms." *Journal of Counseling Psychology, 56* (3): 450–60.

15. Bjornsson, A. S., Bidwell, L. C., Brosse, A. L., Carey, G., Hauser, M., Seghete, K. L. M., Schulz-Heik, R. J., Weatherley, D., Erwin, B. A., & Craighead, W. E. (2011). "Cognitive-Behavioral Group Therapy versus Group Psychotherapy for Social Anxiety Disorder among College Students: A Randomized Controlled Trial." *Depression and*

Anxiety, 28, 1034–42. Yalom ID, Leszcz M. (2005). *The theory and practice of group psychotherapy,* 5th ed. New York: Basic Books.

16. Benedek, David M., Friedman, Matthew J., Zatzick, Douglas, & Ursano, Robert J. (2009, March). *Guideline watch: Practice guideline for the treatment of patients with acute stress disorder and posttraumatic stress disorder.* doi:10.1176/appi.books .9780890423479.156498.

CHAPTER 15: Depression and Other Mood Problems

1. Lindsey, B. (2009). "The Prevalence and Correlates of Depression among College Students." *College Student Journal, 43* (4): 999.

2. Benton et al., 2003.

3. Heiligenstein, E., & Guenther, G. (1996). "Depression and Academic Impairment in College Students." *Journal of American College Health, 45* (2): 59.

4. Stansbury, K. L., Wimsatt, M., Simpson, G. M., Martin, F., & Nelson, N. (2011). "African American College Students: Literacy of Depression and Help Seeking." *Journal of College Student Development, 52* (4), 497–502.

5. Stephenson, J. H., Belesis, M. P., & Balliet, W. P. (2005). "Variability in College Student Suicide: Age, Gender, and Race." *Journal of College Student Psychotherapy, 19* (4): 5–32.

6. Lindsey, 2009.

7. Zullig, K. J., & Divin, A. N. (2012). "The Association between Non-medical Prescription Drug Use, Depressive Symptoms, and Suicidality among College Students." *Addictive Behaviors, 37,* 890–99.

8. Forty, L., et al. (2008). "Clinical Differences between Bipolar and Unipolar Depression." *British Journal of Psychiatry, 192,* 388–89.

9. Kwapil, T. R., Miller, M. B., Zinser, M. C., Chapman, L. J., Chapman, J., & Eckblad, M. (2000). "A Longitudinal Study of High Scorers on the Hypomanic Personality Scale." *Journal of Abnormal Psychology, 109* (2): 222–26. doi:10.1037/0021-843X .109.2.222.

10. Cullen, K. R., Klimes-Dougan, B., Muetzel, R., Mueller, B. A., Camchong, J., Houri, A., Kurma, S., & Lim, K. O. (2010). "Altered White Matter Microstructure in Adolescents with Major Depression: A Preliminary Study." *Journal of American Academy Child Adolescent Psychiatry, 49* (2): 173–83.

11. Blue, H. C., Sanfilippo, L. C., & Young, C. M. (2007). "The Pharmacological Treatment of Depression in College Age Students: Some Principles and Precautions." *Journal of College Student Psychotherapy, 21* (3–4): 149–78.

12. Gallagher, R. National Survey of Counseling Center Directors, 2011. International Association of Counseling Services.

13. Lee, C. L. (2005). "Evidenced-Based Treatment of Depression in the College Population." *Journal of College Student Psychotherapy, 20* (1): 23–31.

14. Rottinghaus, P. J., Jenkins, N., & Jantzer, A. M. (2009). "Relation of Depression and Affectivity to Career Decision Status and Self-Efficacy in College Students." *Journal of Career Assessment, 17,* 271.

15. Hirschfeld, Robert M. A. (2005). *Guideline watch: Practice guidelines for the treatment of patients with bipolar disorder.* http://psychiatryonline.org/content.aspx? bookid=28&sectionid=1682557, accessed July 13, 2012.

16. Federman, R. (2011). "Treatment of Bipolar Disorder in the University Student Population." *Journal of College Student Psychotherapy, 25,* 24–38.

17. Ostacher, M. J. (2007). "Comorbid Alcohol and Substance Abuse Dependence in Depression: Impact on the Outcome of Antidepressant Treatment." *Psychiatric Clinics of North America, 30* (1): 69–76.

CHAPTER 16: Psychotic Symptoms

1. Daniel Eisenberg, Healthy Minds Study 2012, University of Michigan, personal communication.

2. Graham, K. M., & Jones, P. B. (2012). "Psychotic Symptoms in Young People without Psychotic Illness: Mechanisms and Meaning." *British Journal of Psychiatry, 201,* 4–6.

3. Varghese, D., Scott, J., Welham, J., Bor, W., Najman, J., O'Callaghan, M., Williams, G., & McGrath, J. (2011). "Psychotic-Like Experiences in Major Depression and Anxiety Disorders: A Population-Based Survey in Young Adults." *Schizophrenia Bulletin, 37* (2): 389–93. Originally published online Aug. 17, 2009. doi:10.1093/schbul/sbp083.

4. Loewy, R. L., Johnson, J. K., & Cannon, T. D. (2007). "Self-Report of Attenuated Psychotic Experiences in a College Population." *Schizophrenia Research, 93,* 144–51.

5. Hegelstad, W. T. V., et al. (2012). "Long-Term Follow-Up of the TIPS Early Detection in Psychosis Study: Effects on 10-Year Outcome." *American Journal of Psychiatry, 169,* 374–80.

6. American Psychiatric Association. *DSM-5 Development.* www.dsm5.org, accessed Sept. 28, 2012.

7. Leweke, F. M., & Koethe, D. (2008). "Cannabis and Psychiatric Disorders: It Is Not Only Addiction." *Addiction Biology, 13,* 264–75.

8. Rodriguez de Fonseca, F., et al. (2004). "The Endocannabinoid System: Physiology and Pharmacology." *Alcohol & Alcoholism, 40* (1): 2–14; APA, *DSM-5 Development.*

9. Khan, M. A., & Akella, S. (2009). "Cannabis-Induced Bipolar Disorder with Psychotic Features: A Case Report." *Psychiatry, 6* (12): 44–48.

10. Scott, J. H., & Cooper, D. L. (2011). "Campus Stalking: Theoretical Implications and Responses." *College Student Affairs Journal, 29* (2): 165–72, 177, 179.

11. Ibid.

12. Hales, R. E., Yudofsky, S. C., & Gabbard, G. O. (2008). *The American Psychiatric Publishing textbook of psychiatry.* Arlington, VA: American Psychiatric Publishing, p. 37.

13. Goulet, K., Deschamps, B., Evoy, F., & Trudel, J.-F. (2009). "Use of Brain Imaging (Computed Tomography and Magnetic Resonance Imaging) in First-Episode Psychosis." *Canadian Journal of Psychiatry, 54* (7): 493–501. Bain, B. K. (1998). "CT Scans of First-Break Psychotic Patients in Good General Health." *Psychiatric Services, 49* (2): 234–35.

14. Fusar-Poli, P., Valmaggia, L., & McGuire, P. (2007). "Can Antidepressants Prevent Psychosis?" *Lancet, 370,* 1746–48.

15. Ibid.

16. Appelbaum, P. S. (2002). "Can a Psychiatrist Be Held Responsible When a Patient Commits Murder?" *Psychiatric Services, 23* (1): 27–29.

17. Hasnain, M., Fredrickson, S. K., Victor, W., Vieweg, R., & Pandurangi, A. K.

(2010). "Metabolic Syndrome Associated with Schizophrenia and Atypical Antipsychotics." *Current Diabetes Reports 10*, 209–16.

18. Allen, S., Amor, L. B., Bedard, A., Desmarais, P.-A., Jourdain, F., & Michaud, D. (2010). "Age-Dependent Metabolic Effects of Second-Generation Antipscyhotics in Second-Generation Antipsychotic-Naïve French Canadian Patients." *Journal of Child and Adolescent Psychopharmacology, 20* (6): 479+.

19. "Atypical Antipsychotic Lurasidone Newly Approved for Schizophrenia." (2011, Dec.). *Brown University Psychopharmacology Update*, pp. 1+.

CHAPTER 17: Emergency Situations on Campus

1. Brown, G. K. (2002). *A review of suicide assessment measures for intervention research with adults and older adults*. Bethesda, MD: National Institute of Mental Health.

2. Center for Collegiate Mental Health, http://ccmh.squarespace.com/ccaps, accessed Jan. 26, 2013.

3. Russell, K. S., Stevens, J. R., & Stern, T. A. (2009). "Insulin Overdose among Patients with Diabetes: A Readily Available Means of Suicide." *Primary Care Companion to The Journal of Clinical Psychiatry, 11* (5): 258–62.

4. Monahan, J., Bonnie, R. J., Davis, S. M., & Flynn, C. (2011). "Interventions by Virginia's Colleges to Respond to Student Mental Health Crises." *Psychiatric Services, 62* (12): 1439–42.

5. Barboza, S., Epps, S., Byington, R., & Keene, S. (2010). "HIPAA Goes to School: Clarifying Privacy Laws in the Education Environment." *Internet Journal of Law, Healthcare and Ethics, 6* (2). doi:10.5580/2d4.

6. Eileen, W. K., Hughes, S., & Hertz, G. (2011). "A Model for Assessment and Mitigation of Threats on the College Campus." *Journal of Educational Administration, 49* (1), 76–94. doi: http://dx.doi.org/10.1108/09578231111102072.

7. Eells, G. T., & Rando, R. A. (2010). "Components of an Effective College Mental Health Service." In Jerald Kay and Victor Schwartz (Eds.), *Mental health care in the college community* (pp. 43–56). West Sussex, UK: Wiley & Sons.

8. Borum, R., Fein, R., Vossekuil, B., & Berglund, J. (1999). "Threat Assessment: Defining an Approach for Evaluating Risk of Targeted Violence." *Behavioral Sciences and the Law, 17* (3): 323–37.

9. Appelbaum, P. (2006). "Law & Psychiatry: 'Depressed? Get Out!': Dealing with Suicidal Students on College Campuses." *Psychiatric Services, 57* (7): 914–16.

CHAPTER 18: Impulse Control Problems, Behavioral Addictions, and Other Problematic Behaviors

1. Grant, J. E., Potenza, M. N., Weinstein, A., & Gorelick, D. A. (2010). "Introduction to Behavioral Addictions." *American Journal of Drug and Alcohol Abuse, 36*, 233–41.

2. Odlaug, B. L., & Grant, J. E. (2010). "Impulse-Control Disorders in a College Sample: Results from the Self-Administered Minnesota Impulse Disorders Interview (MIDI)." *Primary Care Companion to The Journal of Clinical Psychiatry, 12* (2): PCC.09m00842. doi:10.4088/PCC.09m00842whi.

3. Weinstein, A., & Lejoyeus, M. (2010). "Internet Addiction of Excessive Internet Use." *American Journal of Drug and Alcohol Abuse, 36,* 277–83.

4. Ko, C.-H., et al. (2009). "Proposed Diagnostic Criteria and the Screening and Diagnosing Tool of Internet Addiction in College Students." *Comprehensive Psychiatry, 50,* 378–84.

5. Canan, F., Ataoglu, A., Ozcetin, A., & Icmeli, C. (2012). "The Association between Internet Addiction and Dissociation among Turkish College Students." *Comprehensive Psychiatry, 53,* 422–26.

6. Huang, X., et al. (2010). "Treatment of Internet Addiction." *Current Psychiatry Reports, 12* (5): 462–70.

7. Wareham, J. D., & Potenza, M. N. (2010). "Pathological Gambling and Substance Use Disorders." *American Journal of Drug and Alcohol Abuse, 36,* 242–47.

8. Kerber, C. S. (2005). "Problem and Pathological Gambling among College Athletes." *Annals of Clinical Psychiatry, 17* (4): 243–47.

9. Ibid.

10. Weinstock, J., et al. (2008). "College Students' Gambling Behavior: When Does It Become Harmful?" *Journal of American College Health, 56* (5): 513–21.

11. McClellan, G. S. (2008). "What Colleges Can Do about Student Gambling." *Chronicle of Higher Education, 54* (26).

12. Ibid.

13. Weinstock et al., 2008.

14. Wareham & Potenza, 2010.

15. Duke, D. C., Keeley, M. L., Geffken, G. R., & Storch, E. A. (2010). "Trichotillomania: A Current Review." *Clinical Psychology Review* 30 (2): 181–93.

16. Ibid.

17. Christenson, G. A., Pyle, R. L., & Mitchell, J. E. (1991). "Estimated Lifetime Prevalence of Trichotillomania in College Students." *Journal of Clinical Psychiatry, 52,* 415–17.

18. Keuthen, N. J., Wilhelm, S., Fraim, C., & O'Sullivan, R. L. (2000). "Repetitive Skin-Picking in a Student Population and Comparison with a Sample of Self-Injurious Skin-Pickers." *Psychosomatics, 41,* 210–15.

19. Chamberlain, S. R., Menzies, L., Sahakian, B. J., & Fineberg, N. A. (2007). "Lifting the Veil on Trichotillomania." *American Journal of Psychiatry* 164 (4): 568–74.

20. Duke, D. C., Keeley, M. L., Geffken, G. R., & Storch, E. A. (2010). "Trichotillomania: A Current Review." *Clinical Psychology Review, 30,* 181–93. Keuthen et al., 2000.

21. Ibid.

22. Grant, J. E., Odlaug, B. L, & Kim, S. W. (2009). "N-acetylcysteine, a Glutamate Modulator, in the Treatment of Trichotillomania: A Double-Blind, Placebo-Controlled Study." *Archives of General Psychiatry, 66* (7): 756–63.

23. Grant, J. E., & Odlaug, B. L. (2009). "Update on Pathological Skin Picking." *Current Psychiatry Reports, 11,* 283–88.

CHAPTER 19: The Nontraditional Student

1. McCari, D. P., Maples, M. F., & D'Andrea, L. (2006). "A Comparative Study of Psychosocial Development in Nontraditional and Traditional College Students." *Journal of College Student Retention, 7* (3–4): 283–302.

2. Quimby, J. L., & O'Brien, K. M. (2006). "Predictors of Well-Being among Non-traditional Female Students with Children." *Journal of Counseling and Development, 84* (4): 451–60.

3. Dill, P. L., & Henley, T. B. (1998). "Stressors of College: A Comparison of Traditional and Nontraditional Students." *Journal of Psychology, 132* (1): 25–32.

4. Quimby & O'Brien, 2006.

5. Ibid.

6. Bye, D., Pushkar, D., & Conway, M. (2007). "Motivation, Interest, and Positive Affect in Traditional and Nontraditional Undergraduate Students." *Adult Education Quarterly, 57,* 141–58.

7. Herman, D. A., & Davis, G. A. (2004). "College Student Wellness: A Comparison Between Traditional- and Nontraditional-Age Students." *Journal of College Counseling, 7,* 32–39.

8. Gillman, J. L., Kim, H. S., Alder, S. C., & Durrant, L. H. (2006). "Assessing the Risk Factors for Suicidal Thoughts at a Nontraditional Commuter School." *Journal of American College Health, 55* (1): 17–26.

9. JED Foundation. "Understanding and Supporting the Emotional Health of Student Veterans." Online training. www.jedfoundation.org/programs/understanding-and-supporting-the-emotional-health-of-student-veterans, accessed May 27, 2013.

10. United States Department of Defense, Task Force on the Prevention of Suicide by Members of the Armed Forces. (2010). *The challenge and the promise: Strengthening the force, preventing suicide and saving lives: Final report of the Department of Defense task force on the prevention of suicide by members of the armed forces.* Washington, D.C.: Department of Defense.

11. Wood, D. (2012). "Veterans' College Drop-Out Rate Soars." *Huffington Post,* www.huffingtonpost.com/2012/10/25/veterans-college-drop-out_n_2016926.html?utm_hp_ref=college.

12. Rudd, M., Goulding, J., & Bryan, C. J. (2011). "Student Veterans: A National Survey Exploring Psychological Symptoms and Suicide Risk." *Professional Psychology: Research and Practice, 42* (5): 354–60. doi:10.1037/a0025164.

13. USDOD, 2010.

14. Cate, C. A. (2011). "Student Veterans' College Experiences: Demographic Comparisons, Differences in Academic Experiences, and On-Campus Service Utilization." University of California, Santa Barbara. ProQuest Dissertations and Theses 189.

15. Wood, 2012.

16. Krysinska, K., & Lester, D. (2010). "Post-traumatic Stress Disorder and Suicide Risk: A Systematic Review." *Archives of Suicide Research, 14* (1): 1–23. doi:10.1080/13811110903478997.

17. Sinski, J. B. (2012). "Classroom Strategies for Teaching Veterans with Post-traumatic Stress Disorder and Traumatic Brain Injury." *Journal of Postsecondary Education and Disability,* 25 (1): 87–95.

18. US Task Force on the Prevention of Suicide by Members of the Armed Forces, 2010, and Rudd et al., 2011.

19. Welberg, L. (2012). "Traumatic Brain Injury: Brain Trauma in Military Veterans." *Nature Reviews Neuroscience, 13,* 450–51.

20. Ackerman, R., DiRamio, D., & Mitchell, R. (2009). "Transitions: Combat Veterans as College Students." *New Directions for Student Services, 126,* 5–14.

21. Wood, 2012.

22. Hadley, W. M. (2011). "College Students with Disabilities: A Student Development Perspective." *New Directions for Higher Education*, pp. 77–81. doi:10.1002/he.436.

23. Ibid.

24. Bernert, D. J., Ding, K., & Hoban, M. T. (2012). "Sexual and Substance Use Behaviors of College Students with Disabilities." *American Journal of Health Behavior, 36* (4): 459–71.

CHAPTER 20: Models of Treatment

1. Rockwell, W. J. K. (1984). "Brief Psychotherapy with University Students." *Psychiatric Annals, 14* (9): 637.

2. Eichler, R. (2006). "Developmental Considerations." In Paul Grayson & Philip Meilman (Eds.), *College mental health practice* (pp. 21–41). New York: Routledge.

3. Eisenberg, D., & Chung, H. (2012). "Adequacy of Depression Treatment among College Students in the United States." *General Hospital Psychiatry, 34* (3): 213–20.

4. Golden, B. R., Corazzini, J. G., & Grady, P. (1993). "Current Practice of Group Therapy at University Counseling Centers: A National Survey." *Professional Psychology: Research and Practice, 24* (2): 228–30. doi:10.1037/0735-7028.24.2.228.

5. Bjornsson, A. S., et al. (2011). "Cognitive-Behavioral Group Therapy versus Group Psychotherapy for Social Anxiety Disorder among College Students: A Randomized Controlled Trial." *Depression and Anxiety, 28*, 1034–42.

6. Ludwig, D. S., & Kabat-Zinn, J. (2008). "Mindfulness in Medicine." *JAMA, 300* (11): 1350–52. doi:10.1001/jama.300.11.1350.

CHAPTER 21: Treatment Challenges in the University Population

1. Fournier, J. C., et al. (2010). "Antidepressant Drug Effects and Depression Severity: A Patient-Level Meta-analysis." *Journal of the American Medical Association, 303* (1): 47–53.

2. "Options for Mild or Moderate Depression." (2010). *Harvard Mental Health Letter Academic OneFile*. Web. Oct. 30, 2012.

3. Iarovici, D., Parker, S., Rogers, H., & Chaudhary, A. (2008). "A Pilot Study to Examine Potential Differences in Antidepressant Medication Side Effect Profiles in the University Student Population." Poster presented at the American Psychiatric Association Annual Meeting.

4. McCrea, C. E., & Pritchard, M. E. (2011). "Concurrent Herb-Prescription Medication Use and Health Care Provider Disclosure among University Students." *Complementary Therapies in Medicine, 19* (1): 32–36.

5. Bower, K., & Schwartz, V. (2010). "Legal and Ethical Issues in College Mental Health." In J. Kay, & V. Schwartz (Eds.), *Mental health care in the college community* (pp. 113–41). West Sussex, UK: Wiley-Blackwell.

6. McDonald, S. J. (2008). "The Family Rights and Privacy Act: 7 Myths—and the Truth." *Chronicle of Higher Education, 54* (32).

7. Ibid.

8. Ibid.

9. Stanford University, Dean's Leave of Absence Policy, http://studentaffairs.stanford .edu/studentlife/involuntary-leave/policy.

10. Gray, C. E. (2007). "The University-Student Relationship Amidst Increasing Rates of Student Suicide." *Law & Psychology Review, 31,* 137.

11. Zisook, S., Downs, N., Moutier, C., & Clayton, P. (2012). "College Students and Suicide Risk: Prevention and the Role of Academic Psychiatry." *Academic Psychiatry, 36* (1): 1–6. doi:10.1176/appi.ap.10110155.

12. Schwartz, L. J., & Friedman, H. A. (2009). "College Student Suicide." *Journal of College Student Psychotherapy, 23,* 78–102.

13. Ibid. Gallagher, R. National Survey of College Counseling Center Directors, 2011.

14. Garlow, S. J., et al. (2008). "Depression, Desperation and Suicidal Ideation in College Students: Results from the American Foundation for Suicide Prevention College Screening Project at Emory University." *Depression and Anxiety, 25,* 482–88.

15. Stephenson, H., Pena-Shaff, J., & Quirk, P. (2006). "Predictors of College Student Suicidal Ideation: Gender Differences." *College Student Journal, 40,* 109–17.

16. Haas, A., et al. (2003). "An Interactive Web-Based Method of Outreach to College Students at Risk for Suicide." *Journal of American College Health, 57* (1): 15.

Index

Page numbers in *italics* indicate figures and tables.